the
INCONCEIVABLE
TRUTH

the
INCONCEIVABLE
TRUTH

rethinking infertility

Joanna Graham, PhD

AMBASSADOR INTERNATIONAL
GREENVILLE, SOUTH CAROLINA & BELFAST, NORTHERN IRELAND

www.ambassador-international.com

The Inconceivable Truth

Rethinking Infertility

ISBN: 978-1-62020-559-4
eISBN: 978-1-62020-483-2

Cover Design & Typesetting by Hannah Nichols
Ebook Conversion by Anna Riebe Raats

AMBASSADOR INTERNATIONAL
Emerald House
411 University Ridge, Suite B14
Greenville, SC 29601
www.ambassador-international.com

AMBASSADOR BOOKS
The Mount
2 Woodstock Link
Belfast, BT6 8DD, Northern Ireland, UK
www.ambassadormedia.co.uk

The colophon is a trademark of Ambassador

DEDICATION

To Heather and Gillian, my encouragers . . . and the best friends a girl could have.

ACKNOWLEDGEMENTS

My heartfelt thanks to all who shared their stories with me and to those with a 'Shepherds Heart' for all your support, guidance, and advice.

CONTENTS

INTRODUCTION

THE YOUNG WOMAN SPRINTED UPSTAIRS to catch the phone before it rang off. Nearly out of breath, she snatched the receiver. "Hello . . . oh hi, Aunt May, lovely to hear from you."

She always enjoyed her conversations with her only aunt and so snuggled down on the sofa for a good chit-chat.

Aunt May was a kind, jovial woman who always seemed to have a mischievous twinkle in her eye, and it was comforting to hear a familiar voice among all the changes that had recently taken place. The young woman's life was in a good place. She had just moved to a new country to live in a beautiful home with a husband she adored and was about to start a fantastic new job. With her whole life ahead of her, she eagerly anticipated the future.

As she was excitedly chattering about all her plans, Aunt May interjected, "And what about kids? Won't you be thinking about having little ones soon?"

Caught a little off-guard, the young woman laughed good-naturedly. "What? I'm only twenty-three! There's plenty of time for all that in the future, and there's so much I want to do first."

Aunt May kindly probed a little further. "Mm-hmm, that's what a lot of young ones say now, but what if you wake up one day and you're thirty years old and find out either you can't have children or have problems having them?"

Laughing a little louder this time, thinking her aunt ridiculous, the young woman replied, "Don't be silly! That won't happen, and anyway, thirty seems so long away. I can't even imagine being that age right now."

"Just saying," Aunt May replied good-humouredly, "you just never know, and you don't want to leave it too late."

Well, it has been many years since that conversation took place during which time the young woman has often recalled these words. One morning she and her husband did wake up to the realization that it would take nothing short of a miracle for them to have children.

The young woman, now thirty-eight, is me. In this book I want to share some of the journey and transformations that have taken place in our lives since the "what if" of Aunt May's prediction has indeed become our *reality*.

Whether you have experienced primary or secondary infertility or are a family member, friend, or pastor of someone going through this trial, all would agree—infertility sucks!

Infertility at any stage can be the most soul-destroying experience in life, wrecking marriages and crushing spirits in its unyielding wake. Almost a taboo subject, it can leave one with more questions than answers in addition to confusion about where to turn for advice. It's often very easy (and extremely annoying) to provide a "textbook biblical answer" without reconciling the feelings of the heart with the thoughts of the mind and the leading of the Holy Spirit. But that's not real life. In this book I want to be honest with you about the realities of infertility for the Christian and share some *truth* of what it is to be unable to *conceive*. There is a massive difference between what we are often advised to think and feel, and the realities of the experience. I hope this book will encourage you to be honest with each other and with the Lord.

Having been on this road for the last seventeen years, I have encountered many women and couples, young and old, who have experienced the sorrow of infertility, but far fewer who have come out the other side to a place of peace and joy. I have become convinced that much of the reason for this is because their counsel has not been rooted in Scripture or in Christ. God has so much to teach us from His Word for this season of our lives, and when His Word becomes alive to us, there is nothing more exciting. Therefore, much of what I write is my musings on the Scriptures. God's Word is more powerful than anything I could ever say, so I pray that it speaks to you as it has to me.

As a culture, and perhaps more so as Christians, we're just not very good at discussing infertility. No one really wants to ask questions because they think it might be too painful for you or just plain awkward for them. By sharing some of our own experiences of how God led us through some of the difficult issues associated with infertility, I hope to help you to make God-honouring decisions and understand more the place of infertility in your life.

I do not presume to provide all the answers, but my prayer is that, as you read this book and confront some of the same issues we did, you will see that even infertility can be an amazing opportunity for us to display God's Son—and not ours—to the world.

Every individual couple's journey and experience will be different and unique to them. It's impossible for me to cover every aspect of infertility in a person's life, but hopefully our story will provide a starting point for you to have the confidence to question how you really feel, to help you communicate with each other, and to make Christ-honouring choices based on the Scriptures. I pray you will be comforted as I share what God has taught us from the Bible that helped us then and continues to help us now in how we regard our infertility.

Above all, my prayer is that through your hurt, this book may help the eyes of your heart to be lifted above your problems and refocused on Jesus.

I want you to know, brothers, that what has happened to me has really served to advance the Gospel.

~ Philippians 1:12

CHAPTER 1

OUR JOURNEY

IT WAS DURING MY FIRST year at university that my life crossed paths with the most amazing guy I know. Our eyes met across the pool table in a smoky student bar, and that was it! He had come from Northern Ireland to study in Scotland. We seemed like the perfect match and wanted the same things out of life. While we worked hard, we also had a lot of fun together. He got on so well with all my friends and family that in no time he had become a normal part of our lives and home. It wasn't long before I fell completely head over heels in love with Stephan. Everything was amazing!—or so it would seem.

Neither of us were Christians. The entire time we had been together, so many dear friends and family had been praying for us. We'd been together about a couple of years when the Holy Spirit really started to convict me of my sin. Soon a raging battle was being fought in my mind. I desperately wanted to surrender to Jesus but also wanted to marry this amazing guy, and Jesus was asking me to choose.

By that time, Stephan had taken a job that was about a three-hour journey from my parents' home. As usual after spending the weekend with us, he traveled back to his own place that Sunday evening. I cannot remember the reason why, but that particular weekend, he'd had to leave a little earlier than normal.

With nothing else to do that Sunday evening, I decided I might as well go to church. That night the pastor spoke—as if only to me—of this spiritual battle. He said, "There's someone here who right now has a battle going on in their head, and Jesus is pulling you one way and the world the other, and you must choose!"

I was almost dumbstruck but resolved that night to give my life over to Jesus, even if that meant leaving the man I loved behind. I had no idea how I was going tell Stephan I couldn't marry him. I dreaded the conversation but knew I couldn't disobey Jesus in this.

Unbeknown to me, that very same night, Stephan was also having an encounter with God at the other end of the country. He had been going through the very struggle I had and didn't know what to do about it. Traveling home that evening, he too became strongly convicted of his need for Jesus as his Saviour. Almost not wanting to deal with it then, he turned on the radio for a distraction. This was so unusual for Steph; he never listens to music in the car. As the music blared out, the words in a random pop song, "this could be our last chance," shook him to his core. In that moment he pulled his car over to the roadside and gave his life to Christ.

It was close to midnight when we both surrendered our lives to Christ, on the same night but at opposite ends of the country, each of us unaware of what the other had done.

Sometimes, God will give us the desire of our heart, but we must first surrender those desires to Him. Praise the Lord, we were prepared to give each other up for Him, and by His mercy He gave us back to each other. We were married in September 1997, and Jesus most definitely has been the glue as we are learning more and more to try and make Him our goal.

I fully expected there to be some challenging times throughout the course of our marriage but never expected the first of them to come so soon. Two days after our honeymoon, Steph had an accident at work and smashed up his back and lost the power in his right leg. After weeks of numerous examinations, we were told it was likely he would spend the rest of his life in a wheelchair.

As you can imagine, at this point there was absolutely no thought of us having children. It was all we could do to look after each other. I was to give up my studies to become his full-time caregiver and do what I could to help him continue his work from home as much as his health would allow.

For the next two years my focus was to take care of Steph as we tried to figure out what direction our lives would go. There would be constant hospital appointments and scans and physiotherapy three to four times a week. Never mind walking, he was unable to dress or even wash by himself. Many times I would come home to find him lying on the living room floor, unable to get up after having tried to get off the couch by himself.

He had decided that since it looked like he would never be able to drive again, he would enroll in a master's program to give him more options for future employment. I drove him to class every day and waited in the car until he was finished so I could help him back out. I remember being called into his class to lift him off the floor after he'd fallen off the chair and couldn't get back up. It took the both of us to do even the most simple of tasks.

After about eighteen months, by God's mercy and everyone else's amazement, Steph started to gradually get better. The nerve damage wasn't as severe as first thought, and feeling began to return to his leg. Little by little he regained his strength. With much perseverance and physio, he was able to walk with the help of braces to hold up his feet and crutches to support his arms. By the time he graduated, he was able to walk up onto the stage completely unaided to claim his certificate, with only a slight limp giving away his pain. As you can imagine, we were thrilled with the extent of his recovery. While we knew he would never be completely okay again and would always have some level of pain, we both had an attitude of mind that we would make up for lost time and grab life with both hands.

Just about this time, my best friend (and sister-in-law) became pregnant with their first son. We laughed and celebrated together and joked about how fun it would be if we were pregnant together and our kids could grow up together just as we had done.

Steph and I had nothing more than a brief chat about having one of our own and decided, very casually, "if it happened, it happened; if not, no biggie."

Well, nothing did happen, but to be honest, we hardly even noticed as we were so busy with life. Right after graduation, Steph was head hunted by a company in Northern Ireland for a position he would be able to do with minimum irritation to his health issues. We agreed to go for one year and then re-evaluate our situation.

From our very first week in NI, many people asked us when we were going to "start our family." I actually found it a little comical that so many people seemed to think this was even a priority for us. While I admit fleeting thoughts may have popped into my mind from time to time that "kids still hadn't happened," I certainly did not dwell on them. We were quite content to enjoy life together, just the two of us. Anyway, I wasn't going to hang about waiting for it to happen and went back to study for my own master's.

My main interests were microbiology and embryology, and so I applied for the position of embryologist in the reproductive technology department of the nearby hospital. I was so excited when the interview panel indicated that they were very happy with the way the interview had gone. I left the room full of hope at the prospect of what might be a dream career for me.

I hadn't even made it back to the car before the Holy Spirit knocked on my heart and started to convict me of being involved in this profession. I was so confused, and by the time I arrived home, I thought I was going nuts. By that evening I was convinced this was not what God wanted of me and that if I pursued this career, I would be asked to do things that He did not want me to do. I knew I should withdraw my application and never considered that only a few years down the line, I would be asking the same difficult questions, only as a patient and not an employee.

As the months rolled on, and with the passing birth of each niece, nephew, or friend's baby, we really started to wonder if there was something wrong with us. Maybe I was just more aware of them now, but there seemed to be so many comments and questions from relatives and friends about why we weren't having any children. While such remarks hadn't seemed to bother me much before, they had now become very hurtful and seemed to pierce my heart in a new way. It was as if every decision we made was being judged in light of our having kids. To be honest, it was a bit hurtful to have people think we were living for only our own interests and future, when all the time we were starting to experience the real pain of infertility.

With no kids on the horizon and Steph having now gained permanent employment in NI, we had to think about where our future was headed and what I was going to do with my life. There was definitely a growing fear in us now that it was highly likely that we had a serious infertility problem, and although we prayed about it off and on, we did not really seek the Lord's guidance or ask Him for His help. I think there may have been even some denial about how serious our situation was as we kept believing we were still young enough to put it off to another time in the future.

I had decided that, should I not be able to pursue a career in embryology, I would love to be involved in scientific research within the area of microbiology. That year I was offered and accepted a PhD studentship in microbiology. Again I was amazed at much of the reaction from close friends and relatives to my decision to continue studying.

"Oh how long will that take? Will you still be able to have a family while you do this? Does this mean you won't be able to have any kids for the next three years? Why are you so career-minded? Don't you think you are being a bit selfish?"

In reality, we were not completely career-minded at all, but what other option did we have? We did not have any kids for me to be the "stay at home mom" that everyone thought I should be. The truth was, I wasn't choosing one life path over another. I didn't have the privilege of having that choice.

These comments hurt now more than ever. It was becoming increasingly more difficult to watch the pregnant bellies of my friends and relatives as they experienced the joy and miracle of growing life and adding to their families. We were expected to visit the hospital when a wee one was born and be all happy with congratulations. When we would arrive, it would always be the same: "Oh, when are you guys going to have one?" or "Well, does this not put you in the notion?"

Occasions such as birthday parties, family gatherings, and Mother's Days at church were very difficult and yet the smile had to be on our faces for fear of making anyone else feel bad or uncomfortable. Sometimes I would feel physically sick or found it difficult to breathe if I thought about it too much. I would spend too much time in the shower crying with a deep sense of sadness and loss for something we had never had.

I could say that we were really strong Christians who never questioned God about why this was happening to us. But that would be lying, because we weren't. Many, many times I accused God, "Why us? What have we done to deserve this?"

For the time being anyway, I reasoned with myself that I should focus on my PhD. We would address our concerns at the end of my studies.

Ironically, the very first week I began my PhD, my new boss, pregnant with her second baby, got to chatting about babies and the right time to start a family. She advised me that in no way should I consider putting off having children for the sake of my studies. Should that happen, she would have no problem working round it. She was perfectly willing for me to do both.

Gosh, if she'd only known.

I don't think I'll need to worry about that, I thought to myself but passed no remarks.

Nearly every year I worked with her, she was pregnant. Each time, the same conversation would come up. My research project took me to various different hospitals and universities, and everywhere I went, there seemed to be someone I was working with who was pregnant.

Are you kidding me, I thought, *these blooming pregnant women—they're everywhere!*

In addition to that, a couple of other students I was friendly with had also gotten pregnant, and so for three years, I was surrounded by pregnant girls my own age who seemed to be juggling kids and work just fine. There was an expectation even then that we "might start a family." One of my colleagues even brought me some of her leftover ovulation sticks, saying, "You can have these, Jo; they work so well, I only needed the one!"

I was then 29 years old and fully aware of the time constraints on my body. I knew the probability of us having a baby naturally was diminishing faster and faster with each passing year.

Publicly, it was almost a comfort to be able to use my studies as an excuse for not starting a family. Everyone just assumed that we both wanted careers. I know many thought we were being very selfish in our outlook to life. All the while, in private, we were experiencing a sadness and confusion that was reinforced as we were reminded every month that I wasn't pregnant.

It was also around this time that we experienced what I can describe only as a weird type of loneliness. Although we had many good friends, there just seemed to be a silence surrounding the subject of infertility. We felt there was no one we could turn to who would not only understand but would be able to give us sound biblical counsel. Perhaps we were not looking in the right places, but there just seemed to be a real lack of Christian advice or guidance. There were a few times I tried to bring it up in conversation with others, but the response would always be one of two; either they would feel very awkward and didn't know what to say so said nothing, or they would be dismissive and hurtful with comments like "well, maybe you're just not doing it right" or "you just never know; don't give up hope." Therefore, for the most part, we kept all our struggles to ourselves and let people assume what they would.

By the time I had started my post-doctoral research position, Steph and I decided that if nothing happened in the next year, we would take a year off work, go travelling round the world, and seriously discuss what we should do about having or not having any children.

Nothing did happen in that next year, and so we bought a world map and planned the trip of a lifetime. We gave notice on our jobs, sold our house and cars, and organised our travel tickets. It was all set up. We were so excited to be going round the world, a perfect distraction and "consolation" for all our disappointment and emptiness.

It was the week before we were due to pay the final deposit on our tickets, after which all our money would be non-refundable. We were out for dinner with friends, discussing all our plans, when we got the phone call.

"Stephan, there's something wrong with your dad."

We hurried home to find he'd collapsed on the bathroom floor and had to be rushed to the hospital. He had suffered a severe brain clot, and his life was hanging by a thread.

I'm ashamed to say it, but at the time I thought, *Oh no, you've got to be joking! What about our trip?* I couldn't believe this was happening. There was no way we could go and leave Stephan's dad and mom. We were all they had. I cannot lie; I was completely gutted.

Stephan continued on with his employment, and I was left to look after his parents. His mom's physical and mental health was fragile enough without the added pressure of his dad. So while Steph was working, it was up to me to visit Tom throughout the day in hospital and take care of Steph's mom at home.

Tom's clot had left him very confused, and although he didn't even know who I was, he wanted me to be there with him all the time. As he very slowly improved, he was required to do physiotherapy every single day. This he completely refused to do unless I was there.

One evening while visiting, I chatted with his consultant who was friends with a former colleague of mine with whom I'd just had a paper published. We had discussed some of my work, and I was reminded that only a couple of months previous, I'd had opportunities to work in the area of my research in a number of different countries. I looked over at Tom and sighed as I noticed his catheter bag needed changing. I went over to the bed and was about to unhook his bag to change it when I slid to the floor at the end of his bed and started to cry. I wept in despair that this was where my life had led me. As I sat there on the hospital floor, holding this bag for an old man that I didn't really have a close relationship with, I cried out to God in frustration.

Is this what I gave up my career for? I've no job, no house, no trip, and we can't even have any kids!! This is so unfair, Lord, what am I doing here? I hate this and feel like I just want to walk away for good!

That night changed my life and has affected so much of who God is making me into since then.

It wasn't an audible voice, but it was the next clearest way I believe the Holy Spirit can "talk to you." Very clearly He told me, "Jo, I do have a plan for your life, but right now I need you to learn to be a servant, and as you sit there holding that bag, you must be prepared to do this for Me. Right now I want you to look after Tom, but for Me."

I'll never forget that night and many times since then, when I feel I'm entitled to more of what this world has to offer, including children, I've been reminded of that moment. Then I ask God to give me that servant's heart for Him first and be in the place He wants me to be.

For the next six months, I watched as the life I had known slipped down the drain, and a new one started to emerge in me. God was changing me every day that I went into that hospital to care for my father-in-law who didn't even know who I was. Every time I had a "wobble" and wanted to pack my bags for a "better" life abroad, God reminded me of a verse in Genesis 26 when Isaac wanted to escape the famine in his own country. He wanted to go to Egypt where it seemed like life would be better and where he wouldn't have to experience any discomfort. God said to Isaac (and to me), "Do not go down to Egypt, live in the land where I tell you to live, stay in this land . . . and I will be with you and I will bless you" (Gen 26:2a-3a, NIV).

As I conceded to sticking it out in NI, God started to show me that I had to learn to want what He wanted for me, which was not necessarily what I wanted. How He has grown this desire in me and Steph has been pivotal in how we have coped through the latter stages of our infertility journey.

After about seven months, we brought Tom home. As he slowly continued to improve, Steph and I were able to move out and have some space to think about what to do next. All our previous plans had been turned upside down, and they were about to take another turn that we could not have expected.

Within a few weeks of our moving out from looking after Steph's parents, circumstances arose that meant two little nephews moved to NI to live with us. I know many people looked on this arrangement as our having the children we'd been waiting for, but this was not the case at all. We loved these kids so much and wanted to help them in any and every way we could, but we never wanted to take the place of their mom. These were our precious little nephews and we loved them unconditionally, but we were aunt and uncle, not mom and dad.

I used to think it was funny when people would say, "You love them like they were your own," when we had no idea what that was like. How did we know, when we didn't have "our own" with whom to compare? Nonetheless, the boys very quickly settled into life in NI.

By now I was 32 years old and fully aware of my body's time limitations. We knew that if we were seriously going to investigate this further, now was the time to do it, so after much prayer, we made an appointment to visit the doctor. Our journey down this road took us all the way to undertaking full-blown reproductive intervention techniques and experiencing all the turmoil those procedures entail. (I cover this part of our journey in detail in chapter 2 on ART and share with you some of the pitfalls and questions that we encountered and which we feel are vital for all Christian couples to explore.)

Throughout this whole journey though, we had told no one. This was in part because we were very private in certain areas of our lives, and there was definitely a little self-preservation going on. In addition, without exaggeration, nearly all of our friends were going through really difficult times of their own; rightly or wrongly, we felt we couldn't burden them with our problems as well. If nothing else though, it forced us to talk to each other and to Jesus more and more just to get through each day. Sometimes hourly, we had to take our aching hearts to Jesus and be honest with Him and each other about how we were truly feeling.

Throughout so much of our story, Jesus has shown us over and over that as we learn to lean on Him, He will use much of what had seemed so painful to heal us without curing us.

Through this journey, Christ has changed our hearts and given us treasures that we wouldn't swap for anything. He has taught us through His Word to learn to want what He wants for us and to make Him our deepest desire. Honestly, I'd go through this "fertility furnace" a million times over rather than go through life settling for less and never knowing Christ the way I do. I don't believe that there is anything this world could offer me that I'd trade for what He is to me, and if this is the journey He needed to take me on to get me there, it is so worth it. It's like He opened my eyes to see more of the depths of His love for me and gave me a love for Him, His people, and the lost that I don't know I would've had otherwise.

My prayer is that as you read and connect with some of our experiences, you will encounter Jesus in a new way—if not for the first time. It is my heart's desire that you will find Him to be the main focus of your heart and that your love for Him will help you to make choices that will honour Him and lead you to a place of peace and worship.

CHAPTER 2

THE "ART" OF CONCEPTION

"GOOD LUCK! IVF FOR CHRISTIANS is a freaking hard topic to talk about!"

You may knowingly chuckle at the above quote, taken from a discussion forum on Christian fertility, but it is true and largely typical of many comments left on such boards by Christian women and men. As controversial as they are, I have noticed that infertility treatments seem to be one of the first things that people want to talk about. Some of the most difficult questions Christian couples face surround this highly sensitive topic of Assisted Reproductive Technologies (ART), and the often conflicting "advice" from highly respected biblical scholars, medics, and scientists can at times seem so confusing.

While some of these advisors would express grave concerns over the practice of reproductive intervention and err on the side of advising against utilizing it at all, others would be strong advocates of many of the technologies available and encourage their application. Therein lies a dilemma for many Christian couples when trying to understand a whole constellation of issues about which there are seemingly numerous perspectives. Many times, it can seem overwhelming for the Christian couple to try and navigate their way through these very complex moral and medical issues, and so they end up deciding it is simply too difficult to decipher what they *can* do from what they *should* do. I hope to clarify some of these queries and provide you with a very practical and biblical understanding of some of the most pertinent issues surrounding ART.

We don't need to go through exactly the same experiences in order to learn from each other. Therefore, it's important that we listen to the invaluable knowledge and wisdom of others who themselves may not have experienced infertility. Having said that, I admit to having felt just a little pang of disappointment in the realization that their understanding of this particular part of our journey is limited by their own personal experience. I think there may be some importance to this because I believe the combination of emotional, hormonal, physical, and often spiritual turmoil involved is arguably unique to this situation in life. The merging of an individual's mind, body, and spirit will inevitably influence their choices and desired outcomes in this area.

During this time of your life, you may find yourself at your most vulnerable—emotionally, mentally, physically, and spiritually—and for this reason alone, the Christian couple experiencing and anticipating reproductive intervention should pause and consider this part of their journey very carefully. It's important for you to know that as we explore some of these questions I myself have wrestled with issues surrounding ART and I am in no way sitting in judgement of anyone trying to work through these same difficulties. Having walked this path, I fully understand your pain and the strength of your natural longings for a child.

This chapter isn't meant to be a comprehensive manual on reproductive technology or even an in-depth bioethical assessment on the subject. My desire is to try and present the science and ethics in a very simple way so you will have at least a place to begin answering some of your questions. The Bible is not a reproduction textbook and thus many of the particular issues involved can be difficult to resolve. Therefore, what I put forth is demonstrative of my own personal convictions based upon what I believe the Scriptures teach about these things.

Let me just say that the moral status of every child, regardless of how they were conceived, is never and should never be in question. Every single child is born in the image of God and should be celebrated as the precious son or daughter that he or she is.

I want to take you on some of our ART journey, highlighting key lessons and experiences that will hopefully help you and give you the confidence to make sound biblical choices for your own circumstances. Even though the specifics of your treatments and procedure will be different from mine, you may be able to apply some general principles of what God taught us as you embark on your own roller coaster ride of ART.

THE HEAD AND THE HEART

As couples and individuals seeking to "walk in a manner . . . fully pleasing to Him," we must ask ourselves one of the most obvious questions in relation to ART: where in terms of our Christian convictions do we draw the line between what we would or would not be willing to do in our pursuit of producing a child?

In order to arrive at wise and God-honouring conclusions about how/if we should be involved in ART, we must consider all of the issues in terms of both *the mind*, on an intellectual basis, and *the heart*, engaging our emotions and desires. I believe it is unwise, if not reckless, for the Christian to divorce the mind from the heart when approaching this subject, because how we "set our minds"—along with being "led by the Holy Spirit" (Rom. 8)—will determine what we do with our physical bodies.

Even before we consider undertaking any type of reproductive therapy, we need to give ourselves adequate time to consider the important moral and scientific questions involved. The decisions that we make based on an intellectual understanding of the procedures and how they are influenced by the motivations of the heart will have a huge effect on what we will do with our bodies.

Therefore, it is imperative that, even at the earliest stages in your ART journey, the heart's desire be aligned with the intellectual reasoning of the mind. If these two aspects are in conflict, you are in danger of allowing this tension to lead you in a path that would not honour God.

For example, if you do not equip yourself with at least a basic understanding of the science behind the technology, and your heart's longing is first and foremost to have a baby, then you place yourself in the very precarious position of handing responsibility for the medical decisions over to someone else, most likely your fertility doctor. The implications of such a judgement can be huge.

On the other hand, if the mind directs you to make intellectual choices that appear to be God-honouring but are not borne out of a heart that seeks to put Him first but where again the deepest desire is to have a baby, then this will create inner friction that has the potential to breed long-term resentment and blame.

If you don't ever bridge the gap between the head and the heart, there is a danger you will carry your frustration and anger throughout the rest of your life. I have witnessed this in women in their 50s and 60s who are still living with bitterness because the past decisions they made were not in concordance with the true longings of their hearts. This divergence in their spirits has never been resolved to bring them to a place of peace and contentment. If the right motivations of the heart do not influence the decisions of the mind and vice versa, then they will never lead us to a place of fulfilment and worship but will create an opportunity for lingering pain and hardness of heart to take root.

I am convinced that only when a couple has begun to confront such issues and has decided to make their truest desire to put the Lord first in all these decisions are they ready to deal wisely with the information about the technical procedures. This will have a significant bearing on the very practical choices you must make about the type of reproductive interventions you may participate in. It's so important we don't miss this step. We can't talk about the pros and cons of ART on a scientific basis before we examine the condition of our spiritual heart first.

This was one of the very first lessons that God taught us in our ART journey and continued to reinforce it at various stages along the way. As we explore this subject, try to constantly consider these issues both in terms of the mind and the heart.

At 32 years of age and married for 11 years, we both knew that if we were going to investigate our infertility further, we probably shouldn't leave it much longer. The decision to go see the doctor for the first time was not an easy one for us. My background as a biological research scientist had stirred in me many questions and reservations concerning the actual procedures involved in ART, and I knew that before we ventured down this path, God was really going to have to prepare our hearts and give us very clear guidance. As a couple we talked at length about how far we would be prepared to go. We prayed individually and together for weeks before we decided to approach our doctor.

It was during these particular weeks that God began to bring to our thoughts a whole different set of questions that were going to be far more important for us to address than those surrounding the technicalities of ART. These were questions relating to where our hearts were with Jesus and with each other. Questions such as:

What would we do or how would we feel if the investigations found that we definitely couldn't get pregnant? Wouldn't it just be better not to know for sure? Then at least we would always have a little hope, as in "you just never know."

Would opening "Pandora's box" create a whole new dynamic in our marriage? How might we feel as individuals and as a couple if we found out that we were the one with the problem and the other person was perfectly fine? Would we feel that we had let our partner down? Would they secretly blame us, and would resentment or bitterness grow if we knew?

If the answer is definitely no to pregnancy, how would we cope with that?

These are very difficult questions that many Christian husbands and wives ponder in their hearts but never truly acknowledge to each other or before God. We frequently hear how the Christian couple should view infertility as a condition to be borne equally by both spouses; the couple is encouraged not to view it in individualistic terms or as being the fault or problem of just one. While this is right and good advice to heed, the reality of the situation can sometimes be very different. We find it safer to say the "right thing," even if it's the opposite of our true thoughts and feelings. I have witnessed so many Christian couples who seem to find it difficult to communicate with each other about the simple things in life, never mind these deep, soul-searching issues. Indeed I know of couples who decided against any medical investigations for fear their relationship would not withstand the impact; should one partner find out they were to "blame."

As Stephan and I openly and honestly discussed these things and purposed to reassure each other that no negative feelings would be allowed to develop, we actually had no real way of knowing how our hearts would respond when the time came. Therefore we spent much time in prayer together, inviting Christ into our conversations and asking for His protection and guidance over our hearts and marriage. Don't get me wrong, we had a very strong, loving, and happy marriage with no preexisting seeds of frustration or bitterness, but these were deep questions of life that we had not fully faced until this point. We felt an extra need to guard our hearts. We asked Christ to keep our hearts sweet toward Him and for each other, no matter what outcome the medical investigations might reveal.

I realize that our being married for a longer time may have made it a little easier for us to address these difficult questions together than it is for those of you who are being confronted with these issues after a shorter amount of time. Therefore, I would urge you both to pray for each other before engaging in these conversations and ask the Holy Spirit to guide your heart and your words as you grow in trust with one another.

As we sought to do this, Christ very gently made it so clear to us that no matter what we chose to do, in all our decisions He had to come first. It was imprinted then on our hearts that first and foremost, our priority had to be to honour Jesus above all else.

So with this in mind, we made the decision to go see the doctor and explore our options. Walking in her door, I prayed, "Lord, let me honour You in this, and help me make the right choices." From that day on, I prayed the same prayer before each appointment. I was almost scared not to pray this or depend on Christ to make my decisions for me. There were moments of weakness where, had He not been in control, I'm sure I would have made choices based on what I wanted rather than what I believed would honour Him. I knew I would have to hang on to this if I was really going to surrender my will to His. This was so painful at times and to outsiders it often didn't make any sense. This became very apparent to us during our first visit to our fertility specialist.

I remember how quickly the consultant called us into her office in almost a "hurry up, my time is money" kind of way. No sooner had we sat down than she stated the exact procedure we would be undertaking before proceeding to push what seemed like a thousand forms in front of us to countersign without any explanation of what the procedure entailed or whether we were ready to undergo the treatment. After all, she had a waiting room full of people outside, and it felt like she couldn't get us out of her office quickly enough.

I was boiling inside. With tears stinging the back of my eyes, I quietly put down the pen on her desk, looked her in the eyes, and calmly said, "No, I'm not okay with this. I have many questions and don't want to sign or agree to anything until all my concerns have been addressed."

We explained to her what we were and were not willing to consent to. This ranged from how much we were willing to take part in research, to how many eggs we would allow to be fertilized, to how many embryos we would want implanted, should they occur.

She looked at me, with the most beautiful eyes I'd ever seen, like I had two heads. Complete confusion was written across her face. She tried to explain to us that what we had just proposed made no sense in terms of achieving the highest chance of obtaining a positive result from this procedure. She couldn't understand why we would go through with the procedure at all if we were not going to maximize the opportunity.

We gently explained to her that based on our Christian convictions, this was the only way we could go through with the procedures, and if she didn't feel it would be worth it, then we were happy to withdraw fully from the treatment plan. Although she agreed to our requests, she made it very obvious that she was not happy about our conditions. She probably thought we were wasting her time. From an unbeliever's perspective, I could completely understand why she might feel we were not taking full advantage of the technology and were perhaps even being a little selfish or unreasonable in our approach.

Driving home, Stephan and I were not only left a little shocked by what had just taken place, but we became very concerned about how easy it could be for Christians to agree to procedures they did not fully understand. Had I not had a science background, I too would have struggled to ask pertinent questions or understand exactly what we were agreeing to. This is why I believe it is so important for Christian couples to be equipped with at least a basic knowledge about such treatments. The decisions you make at this stage can have a profound effect on your own life as well as have the potential to be a powerful testimony to those around you.

Now let's look at some of these individual fertility procedures and discuss the science behind them. This is in no way an exhaustive list, but it includes the more common therapies, and many of the same principles we apply to them can also be applied to most others.

Remember though, as we consider these technologies, we need to be engaging both our minds and our hearts.

THE ART OF CONCEPTION

Perhaps the first question we need to be asking ourselves is "how do we honestly feel about even asking these questions in the first place?" Do you even want to investigate these issues further and become better informed, or do you not care too much as long as the outcome is the one you want? After all, if my computer breaks down, I'm not even slightly interested much less care what the engineer does to resolve the problem, just so long as it is fixed. That may seem a little facetious, I know, but I have witnessed the same attitude when it comes to couples considering and undertaking reproductive interventions. One of the problems with not familiarizing oneself with the procedures and implications of some procedures is that some prospective parents are hit with moral dilemmas that they hadn't even contemplated until they come up in the treatment room. At that stage, it is often difficult to make sound judgements or indeed be in a position of control to be able to make right and good choices. Therefore, it's a wise thing for the Christian couple to understand these procedures before they even meet with their fertility specialist.

There are many, many forms of ART available, and it's impossible to cover them all in detail here. Therefore, I've selected three of the more common techniques (IVF, ICSI, IUI) that you probably have heard of and can relate to.

IVF stands for *in vitro fertilization,* which involves mature eggs being removed from a woman's ovary to be fertilized by her husband's sperm outside of the body in the laboratory. The egg and sperm sample are placed in close proximity to each other in the same Petri dish to facilitate fertilization in the absence of any physiological obstacles. For example, IVF is normally used to help women who have damaged and/or blocked fallopian tubes (which means the egg and sperm cannot meet naturally); endometriosis; unexplained infertility; or in cases where the quality of the man's sperm is poor. A few days after fertilization occurs, the resulting blastocyst (embryo) is placed back into the uterus through a process referred to as *embryo transfer*.

The treatment of IVF is normally performed in five different stages as follows:

Ovarian Stimulation – This is performed with the objective of collecting more than one egg from the ovary to increase chances of embryos being formed and selected for transfer. Approximately every 28 days in a woman's normal menstrual cycle, several follicles (little fluid-filled sacs each containing a single egg) start to grow in the ovaries. However, under normal circumstances only one of these follicles grows large enough to release its egg, a process known as ovulation. Through administration of hormone treatment, it is possible to manipulate the body in a way that allows many follicles to develop at the same time. These hormones are usually given in the form of nasal sprays and injections and will often result in the maturation of between 5-10 follicles.

Monitoring of Egg Development – Throughout this process, the ovaries are scanned to monitor the size and number of follicles, using a vaginal ultrasound probe. If the progress of the follicles is deemed to be good, then another hormone is given to ripen the eggs before they are collected around 36 hours later.

Egg recovery – It is very normal for a woman to be awake for this procedure; however, they usually require strong pain relief. The egg recovery itself is performed by passing a very long needle along a vaginal scanning probe through the tissue wall into the ovaries. Using a monitor for guidance, the hollow needle is pushed into each follicle in turn and the fluid sucked out and examined under a microscope to check for the presence of an egg, as not every follicle may yield an egg.

Fertilization – If eggs have been successfully recovered, they are then placed in a special fluid in an incubator, and the semen sample is added to the fluid. The laboratory will first concentrate the sample; approximately 50,000-100,000 sperm are added to each egg for optimum opportunity for fertilization to happen. At this stage, it is impossible to predict how many, if any, eggs will be fertilized, so it is normal practice that sperm will be added to every egg recovered.

The occurrence of fertilization can be detected at between 12-18 hours by characteristic microscopic changes in the egg. Only after positive detection confirmed by an embryologist can the final stage of embryo transfer take place.

Embryo Transfer – After being cultured in the laboratory for approximately 2-3 days (differs among clinics), the resulting embryos are ready for transfer to the uterus. A small plastic tube is passed through the cervix and the embryos placed in the cavity of the uterus. It is often the case that not all embryos that have developed will be placed.

If the treatment is successful, then the embryo will implant and attach to the uterine wall, and normal pregnancy will ensue.

ICSI (Intracytoplasmic Sperm Injection) is another very common form of ART and is very similar to IVF, with the main distinction being that only a single sperm is selected and then injected into the center of an egg, using a very fine glass needle. This treatment is usually selected for couples where the semen is not suitable for ordinary IVF. Depending on which country you live in and clinic selected, this type of treatment can be far more expensive due to the more specialised laboratory requirements.

IUI (intrauterine insemination) is perhaps one of the first treatments offered to many couples when they begin to undertake any form of ART. This treatment commonly includes the step of ovarian stimulation in the woman. When the maturation of an egg is detected using vaginal ultrasound scanning, hormones are given to stimulate the release of the egg. When this happens, a sperm sample is deposited using a small catheter that is passed into the womb through the cervix. The prevalence of this technique can vary from region to region; while it's still very common in some countries, in the UK it is now not routinely offered in cases of unexplained infertility, mild endometriosis, or mild male fertility problems where normal conception has not been achieved for at least two years.

THE FACTS VS. THE FEELINGS

Now that we have a basic understanding of some of the more common ART procedures, the next question is "how do we interpret this information in terms of a Christian worldview?" At this stage most Christians will experience a level of conflict in their spirit between their strong desire for a child and the questions of what is right and biblical for them in terms of what reproductive interventions they might engage in. Sometimes the clashing of facts with feelings can become too much to cope with, and trying to work out what is best seems too complicated, so many Christians either ignore the facts and go with their instincts or ignore both and leave all decisions up to their fertility doctor. Many couples check out and leave God in the parking lot as they walk through the doors of the fertility clinic.

This is a really dangerous place to be, whether your doctor is a Christian or not. In these consultations, you are likely to make decisions about matters of life and death that could impact the rest of your life. More than ever, you need to take God with you to every appointment. Don't leave Him in the waiting area; ask Him into the doctor's office and make Him part of the consultation. You are going to need His protection, guidance, wisdom, and strength every time you encounter your

THE "ART" OF CONCEPTION

doctors in what might turn out to be the most vulnerable and difficult season of your life. This is because when it comes to ART, the Christian is being asked profound moral questions in the most intense situation of the consultation room, and the decisions made in those moments can have rippling repercussions on many lives. Many of the bioethical issues Stephan and I endorsed as Christians collided with the attitudes and normal practices of our fertility doctors. The clinician is there for the express purpose of achieving the best result he/she can. The question is, is that or should that be the same reason for you and me?

It is best to come to a conviction about these things before you get into the clinic because when the heat is on, we can easily be persuaded by others. You can be led to trust that "these guys know better than me what they're doing. I have to trust their judgement. After all, they only want what's best for me, right?" This is often far from the truth. Some of these clinics may not be completely altruistic in their practices, but even more significant, these doctors do not know what is best for God's children; only He does. He is the one we need to put our trust in for guidance with these life altering decisions.

Below are some of the most pertinent ethical points surrounding ART that we have the responsibility to consider as we try to navigate through this emotional minefield.

These include some of the more common ethical issues that, in my experience, Christians are most likely to ask about and many of which Stephan and I had to confront along the way. Much of what we call *bioethics*, I call *heart issues*, and so the practicalities of our ART—as influenced by our ethics—was mainly determined by our hearts' desire to honour Christ. We arrived at the convictions we did based upon what we believed the Bible teaches, the intellectual reasoning of our minds, and our understanding of the character of our God.

THE QUESTIONS OF LIFE . . .

That very first appointment with our fertility specialist, which I've already shared, caused us to confront a few bioethical hot points that immediately created a level of tension and conflict that followed us throughout the rest of our ART journey. In the space of that 20-minute appointment, we had to make judgement calls on issues surrounding the origin of life and the question of when life begins; the distinction between the function of an individual cell and that of an embryo; and the embryo's role within embryonic/cell research. We were required to confront issues about the actual technology used, the implications of artificially manipulating our biological systems, and the perceived payoff between financial input and best probable outcomes. All this within 20 minutes and under the pressure of being persuaded to reconsider from a clinician who "knew best" and had "all the logical answers."

The immediate and predominant question for us to answer was the one of "When does a life become a life?" While relevant to all, perhaps for couples going through IVF or ICSI, the question of when life begins is more fundamental and cannot be ignored for any reason.

This question has long divided and confused our cultures, societies, and individuals. However, from a scientific point of view, the question of when a human becomes a human is often not widely considered to be a controversial one. It is broadly accepted within much of the scientific community as commencing from when a single sperm fuses with a single egg to create a zygote. At this point, all the genetic material and information required for that zygote to grow into a fully functioning, independent adult is contained within those cells. From the point of fertilization, life is on a continuum, seamlessly progressing from the development of the zygote into an embryo, to a fetus, to a child, to an adult, until eventually ending in death.

It could be argued then that if we agree life begins at fertilization, any debate is not so much a scientific one but philosophical, and then the question shifts from being about when a human life begins to when and/or if they deserve any type of care and protection. This introduces the important matter of personhood and the value of a life.

In 1954 Professor Joseph Fletcher proposed that in order for personhood to exist, the human must not only possess a rational nature but also be able to exercise it at the same time. Therefore, by his theory, if the human in the form of an embryo possesses no ability to reason and act upon it, then it cannot be considered a person and in turn should not be afforded the same protection as a rational being.

The Christian couple must ask both of these questions and not only base their answers in science and philosophy alone but also in the Scriptures. The Bible may not talk about IVF or ICSI, but it does have something to say about life from the very Creator of it Himself.

As a Christian, I would wholeheartedly denounce Joseph Fletchers hypothesis and agree with the opposing view that human personhood is defined as one who possesses a rational nature, even if unable to express it at all times. Therefore, all humans are also persons and their life equally valued, and all should be afforded the same level of protection. Indeed, one could propose that those unable to express reason and act for themselves are incredibly vulnerable and therefore should be granted an even higher level of protection, not less.

If you do not believe that each fertilized embryo is indeed a human being made in the image of God, then you must arbitrarily decide at what stage that little embryo becomes a human being. Error at this stage in your thinking can lead to devastating repercussions for their future as well as yours.

The Bible does, however, make it clear that life begins long before a human being is born, and that even at that stage God considers them actual persons. In numerous passages, the Scriptures reference the unborn and demonstrate their personhood—often in personal terms. Below are some of these texts for your own consideration.

"But when he who had set me apart before I was born, and who called me by His grace . . ." (Gal. 1:15).

"Even as He chose us in Him before the foundation of the world . . ." (Eph. 1:4a).

"Before I formed you in the womb I knew you, and before you were born I consecrated you; I appointed you a prophet to the nations" (Jer. 1:5).

"For you formed my inward parts; you knitted me together in my mother's womb. I praise you, for I am fearfully and wonderfully made. Wonderful are your works; my soul knows it very well. My frame was not hidden from you, when I was being made in secret, intricately woven in the depths of the earth. Your eyes saw my unformed substance; in your book were written, every one of them, the days that were formed for me, when as yet there was none of them" (Psalm 139:13–16).

"Listen to me, O coastlands, and give attention, you peoples from afar. The Lord called me from the womb, from the body of my mother he named my name" (Isa. 49:1).

"Behold, children are a heritage from the Lord, the fruit of the womb a reward" (Psalm 127:3).

"In those days Mary arose and went with haste into the hill country, to a town in Judah, and she entered the house of Zechariah and greeted Elizabeth. And when Elizabeth heard the greeting of Mary, the baby leaped in her womb. And Elizabeth was filled with the Holy Spirit, and she exclaimed with a loud cry, 'Blessed are you among women, and blessed is the fruit of your womb! And why is this granted to me that the mother of my Lord should come to me?'" (Luke 1:39–43).

"When men strive together and hit a pregnant woman, so that her children come out, but there is no harm, the one who hit her shall surely be fined, as the woman's husband shall impose on him, and he shall pay as the judges determine. But if there is harm, then you shall pay life for life, eye for eye,

THE "ART" OF CONCEPTION   41

tooth for tooth, hand for hand, foot for foot, burn for burn, wound for wound, stripe for stripe" (Ex. 21:22–25).

If life is therefore on a continuum and God formed us at the start, then He is still in the process of forming us now, not exclusively in a physical sense but in a spiritual one. When we were born again, we became new creations, and He is the one who will continue to form us until finally "we shall be like Him" (1 John 3:2b).

Anyway, it is imperative that you are convinced of the sanctity of life, even in the form of an embryo, so that when doctors come offering you the world, you will be able to stand on your biblical beliefs—even if that means you refuse "the world" to put God's interest above your own.

HOW DO WE WORK SCIENCE AND BIBLICAL CONVICTION INTO OUR OWN ART EXPERIENCE?

As discussed earlier, the normal process of IVF and/or ICSI involves superovulation for the collection of multiple eggs with a view to fertilizing as many as possible. The more eggs fertilized, the greater the probability of acquiring the optimum number of high quality embryos, increasing the chance of pregnancy. It is impossible to determine how many of these eggs, if any, will be successfully fertilized and what the quality of each resulting blastocyst will be. At this stage of the process, it is not the usual practice for the patient to garner any control over the number of eggs deemed suitable for fertilization; these decisions are primarily undertaken by the clinician and embryologist.

Friend, this is one of the crucial stages in your ART journey where I would assert that even though you will most probably be in disagreement with your doctor, you are in fact the one who needs to be making this decision and taking control of how many eggs should be fertilized. We have already established that life begins at the earliest stages of fertilization, when egg meets sperm, and so with every egg fertilized, life has begun.

The individual practices of your fertility doctor will depend on your particular clinic, state, and even what country you live in, but in recent years, the general direction of most practitioners is to move away from the multiple birth scenario to the transfer of just one or perhaps two embryos into the woman. Medical evidence would show that this practice encourages more successful full term pregnancies, reduces miscarriages and loss of preterm fetus, and reduces the risk of medical complications for both mother and baby. In fact, in some countries, it is now required by law that no more than two high quality embryos be transferred at any one time.

Now we begin to understand just why it is imperative that you know how these procedures work before you ever undertake them. This is why you must take Christ into the consultation room with you. If a Christian couple allows for more than two eggs to be fertilized and thereby potentially creates more embryos (lives) than can be physically implanted, they must ask themselves "what happens to these little lives that initially never make it into the uterus."

In the event that they are not transferred into the uterus, there are four other main routes (although there are more) remaining for these little "spare" embryos to go down.

1. The cells of the blastocyst may stop dividing and so the embryo naturally ceases to develop and grow any further. This is a very common occurrence and is normal, especially when the cell quality of the blastocyst is poor. Such a scenario also happens in the normal course of life when conception happens naturally. Many times (up to 70-80% in normal couples) the fertilized egg fails to implant in the uterus and is lost, often without the woman even realizing anything has ever happened.

2. The embryos can be frozen and stored pending transfer into the prospective mother at a later date.

This subject of freezing embryos is perhaps one of the most controversial among Christians who are happy to undergo IVF/ICSI but are not sure of the implications of such a technique. There are more opinions on this practice than I could cover, but a few are reflected in the following comments from Christian women:

> "There is one consent form which I'm struggling with at the moment: should we freeze our embies? My husband is okay with it and the doctor recommends it, but I am not so sure. This is a difficult one."

> "I don't think there is anything wrong with freezing your embryos; they are alive, just sleeping until you're ready for them."

> "In our Christian view, the thing to do would be to freeze your embryos because discarding them would be taking the decision for their survival into our own hands."

> "When you freeze them, they are still alive in a sense, just on hold till you decide you want to use them."

> "We prayed and talked a lot about this issue and we think freezing remaining embryos is another way to embrace life, and either we would use them all or donate them."

> "It really depends on how many children you want."

> "The problem no one talks about is when your family is complete, what do you do with your frozen embryos?"

You can see from these few remarks just how complicated this whole question of "to freeze or not to freeze" is.

Understanding the depth of desire and longing for a child, I do not feel in a position to judge these things and personally know some miracle babies that at one time were precious little frozen embryos. However, the conviction of my heart is that, given the choice, I would encourage the Christian couple to forego the option of retaining "frost-ies," as we say in the TTC world, by not creating them in the first place.

If we have established that life and therefore personhood begins at the moment of fertilization, then we have agreed that as such these embryos should be afforded the same protection and rights as anyone else with the ability to reason. The question then arises that if we follow this logic through, at which stage do we decide that it is not okay to freeze a person? If the technology was available, would we freeze a child at any other age because it suited us, especially if the risks of defrosting them significantly decreased their chance of survival?

I think it is difficult to argue this issue of frozen embryos exactly from Scripture, and the questions of when we are "knit together" and whether this should be allowed to take place outside the womb or not are very deep and difficult to resolve. When it comes to the debate of frozen embryos, I am more persuaded that the argument is not primarily a scientific or bioethical one but rather one of submission and control.

If I am not sure from the Scriptures about how to deal with a very specific problem such as this one, then I need to seek the heart of God to give me a clear sense of peace and confirmation that what I intend to do is what He would want. Stephan and I never received that peace concerning this issue; in fact, the more we prayed about it, the less comfortable we became. In our situation, we had a strong sense that since we had no confirmation from the Lord that creating frosties was the right to do, then we did not want to take the risk that we would be stepping outside of His will for us in this. We felt that in this particular area, for us to hand over all control to God meant giving up any control we may perceive we could have.

I do not believe God ever indicates that He gives us the right or the power to determine how long anyone should live. He is the one to determine the times and places we live (Acts 17:26). Whenever we have so much as a hint that we can control these things, then the problem is not in the practicalities, because God is sovereign, but the problem becomes one of the heart. It's only when we give Him complete control of our hearts as well as our circumstances that we will have an assurance of His approval and support.

3. Any surplus embryos will be destroyed and discarded. Dear Christian, I don't want you to skip over this point as if it is inconsequential. There is no more important point than this to consider. If you believe that life has begun with the creation of these embryos, then by allowing them to be destroyed, you are participating in abortion or—for a better word—murder!

Although we cannot be certain about the exact numbers, it is estimated that over ten million embryos (lives) have been aborted during the course of fertility treatments worldwide. A report produced by the UK fertility regulator HFEA (Human Fertilization and Embryology Authority) revealed that more than 1.7 million embryos created during ART have been thrown away since records began in 1991. Upon reading this report, government official Lord Alton concluded that embryos were being created and thrown away in "industrial numbers." He went on to say, "It happens on a day-by-day basis with casual indifference."

Fellow Christians, this should give you pause for thought and great cause for concern. What these figures demonstrate is that abortion by ART is at epidemic levels and will continue to rise as ever-increasing numbers of couples opt to participate in ART for producing their family.

Do not allow yourself to be "casually indifferent" about these matters. I beg of you, before you ever enter the door of a fertility clinic, recognize that within their walls, there are probably a great deal more lives lost than born. Consider very, very carefully the implications of your actions.

4. Extra, unwanted embryos are submitted for research purposes, where they will be destroyed by law after a period of 14 days.

As a research scientist who depended on donor tissue for cell culture for my own research, I can fully appreciate the desire for clinicians and scientists to request the use of any unused or unwanted "tissue" for research purposes. However, it is important that, when asked to give consent for our "unusable" and "surplus" tissue to be donated, we understand exactly what it is we are and are not agreeing to.

Allowing spare embryos that have resulted from ART to be used for research is firmly, for the Christian, in the same category as abortion. After 14 days, scientific research is no longer permitted legally and all embryos will be destroyed. Given that knowledge alone, I would advocate that, for the Christian, it is in no way acceptable to allow donation of embryos for these purposes.

However, you may also be asked if you would be willing to donate unused *eggs* that may have been collected. Since the egg is just a cell without the ability to survive or develop into a human independently, then it is perfectly permissible to consent to their use in scientific research. I understand this may not be the view of many, and I must reiterate here that these are my personal convictions informed by both my head and my heart.

For us, these decisions were agreed upon during that very first fertility appointment. Equipped with all this information in our heads and biblical convictions in our hearts, Stephan and I explained to our doctor that we only wanted two eggs to be treated, regardless of the amount of eggs recovered, and only under the condition that if both of them were successfully fertilized that they would both be implanted, irrespective of quality. As alluded to earlier, she was not happy; however, this was an easy decision for us to make. It's not just the particular procedure but the top desire of your heart that will be the one that wins out.

It was also during this consultation that we gave consent for any of my spare eggs to be donated to research, while stating that under no circumstances were any embryos to be submitted. Needless to say, it was only because we made a point of going through all these consent forms, reading the small detail, that we were able to discern where we were signing to donate gametes or embryos. Familiar with filling out patient donor tissue consent forms with many of my own study subjects, I was well aware of the importance of reading and understanding anything I signed. However, the impression I received was that, had I not been diligent in this area, I would have been hurried into agreeing to things of which I had little understanding. This is a very stressful and highly emotional situation, and therefore it is so important that you do not allow yourself to be rushed into any decisions, no matter how "silly" you may feel about asking even the most basic of questions.

[Perhaps, just as a side note, it is worth mentioning here that the language used to describe the earliest stages of when an egg fuses with a sperm can itself cause some uncertainty when considering the origin of a life. The use of the words *conception* and *fertilization* can often interchange between fertility clinicians and between clinicians and embryologists. This can be very confusing for the Christian couple trying to make sound judgements, who are left asking "what do these words mean" and "which one should I be most concerned with." The change in definition of these words means that depending on factors such as which country you live in and your doctor's preference, you may be influenced to make unwise choices without even knowing it. Some clinicians will use the term *conception* to describe the implantation of the egg in the uterus, while referring to the exchange of chromosomal information as "fertilization." However, this is not always the case. It is important at the very outset of your experience to ask your clinician and embryologist what exactly they mean when they use these words. You want to be very clear when discussing what you want and why you are asking that of them.]

While I have focused here on some of the more common areas of ART, there are many others that we may encounter, areas for which even more scientific, ethical, and spiritual considerations need to be given. Among them include areas such as embryo adoption/donation; genetic embryo selection and embryo reduction; egg and sperm donation; surrogacy; and use of three-parent embryos. When considering all these complicated technologies, the Christian couple must reconcile the bioethics with the biological science while being led by the Holy Spirit to come to a place of peace and reassurance that in their decisions, God will be honoured.

STRAP YOURSELF IN . . .

So having made these choices, a few weeks later I started the hormone injections. My body didn't know what had hit it. I knew that for the next few weeks, Stephan and I would have to dedicate ourselves to guarding our hearts, especially with my hormonally-induced emotions.

At the end of two weeks of hormones came the morning of the egg retrieval. It was very early in the morning, and I was tired from hiking with my nephew the night before. In a quite matter-of-fact way, I made my way into the fertility center waiting area and sat emotionless for my name to be called. Well, maybe not totally emotionless—I was a little resentful that I'd had to be up before any decent hour of the morning to make this appointment. I sat in the waiting room debating with myself how I would reorganize this whole clinic if I were in charge.

As I was taken through to the treatment room for yet another dignity-robbing procedure, I thought how everything seemed to be so run-of-the-mill and that it was just another day at the office for the staff as they went about their business of examining cells, scanning uteruses, and taking blood. It struck me that I was indeed guilty of much the same thing. My frame of mind was just switch off, get these things over with as little hassle as possible, and get out of here as quickly as I can to start my day as if nothing out the ordinary was happening.

That all changed when the embryologist looked at our notes and questioned again that fact that we only wanted two eggs treated and no more. Again a little frustrated, and I suspected feeling a little sorry for us, he tried to explain that we were reducing our chances very substantially and questioned if we really understood what we were asking. He even went out and brought in another colleague to explain yet again the ratios just in case we wanted to reconsider our options. It would have been so easy to agree; after all, isn't that why we were there

THE "ART" OF CONCEPTION   49

in the first place, to increase our chances of having a baby? As I lay on the bed and prayed, "Lord, help us to honour you in this," I knew that no matter what I felt in that vulnerable place, I had to stick to what I believed was right and explain to them the reasons why.

I could see resignation in the embryologist's face and thought he felt almost pity for me, a committed but nonetheless deluded Christian girl. I felt like I had let this medical team down and in some way had disrespected their expertise and help. Yet I knew if I didn't make these choices, I would regret it for the rest of my life.

After what seemed like an eternity, the phone call came to say both our blastocysts were of the highest quality, and a date was given for the embryo transfer to take place. Again I had to plead my case with the embryologist to implant both and not just one embryo. Pressing the fact it was not normal procedure, he nonetheless agreed. A couple of hours later, it was all over. The medics had done their part. Now it was up to God and my body to do the rest. We would not know for another two weeks if the procedure had been successful and if we were pregnant.

We'd had to cancel a planned holiday due to the timing of the ICSI procedure, so decided that during the two-week wait, we would still head off for a wee break closer to home. The boys were really excited, and the weather was great. All we really wanted to do was spend two weeks relaxing in a lovely hotel and spend the days fishing the rivers and lochs of Ireland.

I was looking forward to it, but my body was still in pain and pumped full of hormones. The slightest thing would set me off in tears. I was constantly fighting to retain my composure and keep a smile on my face in front of the kids. None of my clothes fit properly, and my whole body just seemed out of whack.

The same afternoon we realized our treatment had failed, an old colleague texted to say they were pregnant with their seventh kiddy. While I was genuinely happy for them, I couldn't help but feel like I'd been stabbed in the heart. I wanted to blame all the other stressful situations that had been going on in our lives at the same time for what had happened. This was so unfair. What had we done wrong? But God had clearly allowed this to happen, and not only must we accept it but in some supernatural way remain thankful.

Again daily, sometimes hourly, we had to take our hurt and hearts to Jesus and be honest with him and each other about how we were truly feeling. Over the next few months and years since, as we leaned on him more and more, God used much of what had seemed so painful to heal us without curing us and gave us peace about our next step.

FISHING IN THE WIND

It was a typical Northern Irish summer day (blooming freezing) when I found myself sitting at the harbor for the fifth time that week as I indulged my 10-year-old nephew in his passion for fishing. From inside my car, I watched him standing on the pier, bracing the rain, struggling with his rod and line as it flapped uncontrollably in the wind. I had to admire his determination to brave the weather and unfavorable tides just to try and catch that elusive fish.

The anticipation of just one bite . . . just one nibble, that's what kept him out there. I smiled to myself as the little "frozen snotter" scurried back to the car to borrow my favourite, ten-sizes-too-big Lorenzo MotoGP hoody. He was gearing up just to be able to stay out a little longer in the blustery weather, determined to catch something before we had to head home.

We had been there for hours by this point. I was so uncomfortable, hungry, and dreaming of hot coffee and "defrosting" in front of an open fire. As if on cue, I looked up to see Jack wind in his line and set his rod down on the concrete harbor wall. "Yes," I thought. "We're going home!" Just when I reckoned he'd given up and was folding away his rod, I realized to my dismay that he was only changing his lure! He had that "whatever it takes" look on his face, and I knew then we were going nowhere soon. I have to admit, I held out no hope of him catching any fish that day, but I did love that spirit of a "just maybe" in my little nephew.

As I sat there watching him, it dawned on me that what he was doing was a great illustration of how many couples approach and go through the process of fertility treatment. I think we would all agree that the conditions in our lives are unfavorable as we try to negotiate the intense changes happening in our minds and bodies. We too must brave the emotional winds of change that come with the territory. We must contend with the flapping around of our artificially controlled hormones and on top of all that go through some of the most personal and intrusive physical procedures one could imagine.

We endure all this for the prospect of that elusive catch, believing that eventually at the end of the line, there will be a baby. Most days we have a steely determination and belief that if we persevere, all will work out well. Perhaps we may decide that if one technique isn't working as well as we'd hoped, then we just change the "lure" in the pursuit of this miracle.

For many though going through IVF, there will be no fish caught today and no happy result will arise, no matter the tactic used or amount of positivity mustered. Just as Jack went home that day without any fish, we too can be left with an empty net—or should I say our empty womb. For some couples, the daylight fades and the window of opportunity to keep trying becomes smaller and smaller, until they find that the tide has completely gone out. They couldn't continue to fish even if they wanted to.

But for those of us who still have "a chance," how long and how far do we go down this road in our pursuit of a child?

For Stephan and me, we made the decision not to continue with any more ART cycles for a few different reasons. First, we both felt very strongly that if a child was indeed going to be born to us, then there was no reason why God couldn't bring that about by Himself if He so chose. As much as we had embraced the technology available, it is nothing compared to what our God can do.

Second, we had a strong sense that perhaps we were trying to push open doors that at that time God didn't want to open for us. We were afraid that maybe we were stepping outside His will for our lives and that if we truly believed He knew best for us, then we must be very careful what we asked for.

Another danger associated with ART is that I have seen so many women and men become obsessed and overtaken by their desire to have a baby that IVF/ICSI becomes almost like a drug to the degree that they will keep pursuing until they get a "hit." It reveals the true deep desires of their hearts, believing that if it delivers on its promises, then all their hopes and dreams will be fulfilled. But that's a lie that Christians can fall for just as easily as unbelievers. If we give ourselves over to such things to fulfil our emptiness, we will only be left more broken at the end. If Stephan and I were going to really live out the truth of what God had shown us about Christ being our Living Hope, then we felt we needed to step away from the IVF. It was a choice we made as a way we could display our wholehearted dependence on Jesus and also for the protection of our own hearts and minds.

THE FINAL APPOINTMENT

As we went for our follow up appointments months later, I told my doctor a little of how we felt. With a look of what I think was perhaps puzzlement mixed with admiration, she said, "Jo, this is not the normal response I get. I don't think I have ever had anyone come in here and be as 'sorted' in their heads about all this as you are today." Then, almost as if she'd caught herself, she asked, "Have you spoken to a priest or pastor about this, have they been advising you?"

I'm sure a part of her was a little worried in case we had been negatively influenced by a religious body of some sort, but actually it was my turn to be slightly taken aback.

"No," I replied a little hesitantly as I realized there in her consultation room that most of what had spoken to us and changed us had come directly from reading God's Word. I think this is really when it began to dawn on me that as much as I think counsel in some cases can be invaluable, it must foremost be rooted in the Scriptures.

In the remainder of this book, I want to share with you some of what God taught us from His Word. My heart's desire would be that you too would be blessed and strengthened in your faith for this season of your life.

CHAPTER 3

ANGRY AT THE BIBLE

BE HONEST. HAVE YOU EVER opened your Bible and not liked what you read? I thought so. Me too. I am convinced that one of the most difficult things for many of us Christians to do is truthfully and accurately examine the state of our relationship with God, His Son, and His Word. I suspect many of you would not dare voice aloud your heart's many doubts, frustrations, and even anger toward God, the Bible, and the church. This was certainly true of me for too long before Jesus began to teach me and help me understand more the true essence of His grace.

Having being taught the Scriptures from childhood, I was encouraged to respect them as the ultimate authority for my life without question. For every query I would have, the Bible held the answers; for every struggle I encountered, the Bible would tell me how to get through it; for every moral decision—yep, you guessed it—the Bible offered crystal clear clarification! I'm sure every true Christian would agree with these claims, so why when I turned to the Scriptures now to try and find answers and help for my pain did nothing seem to make sense?

In his book, *Dangerous Calling*, Paul Tripp suggests that "it is dangerous to think that because I know a thing, I am that thing," and just because you can understand and communicate an idea does not mean that you have submitted yourself to it or are living it. He proposes that it is possible to be theologically astute, believing we have "mastered the body of truth," while being simultaneously spiritually immature. What we should be asking instead is this: "To what extent has my life been mastered by this body of truth?"

You see, I reckon this was one of the main reasons for my confusion, because while I knew these things intellectually, they had never really filtered from my head down to my heart. There is a world of difference between intellectual knowledge and believing something at the heart level in a way that impacts and changes your life experientially. This acknowledgement may hold some significance for many of you too when approaching the Scriptures, because you also may accept the Word of God as true and inerrant, and yet it still has little, if any, effect on your life when seeking guidance about infertility. I believe there is such a danger that when seeking wisdom for these issues, we merely "think" our way through the Scriptures without engaging our hearts. Or conversely, we are unable to think rightly because we are ruled by our emotions.

This was true of us as a couple and for me especially. I became resentful and angry about what I was reading in God's Word. A mixture of pride, arrogance, and a misunderstanding of God's character created a swirling pot of skewed emotions that simmered in the slow cooker of my heart. I did not want to accurately examine the true state of my relationship with God and felt guilty about my intense feelings of frustration at His Word.

But, little by little, the Holy Spirit has been so kind to me in revealing more and more the true nature of the Father's heart and the wonderful truth of His Words. The freedom that comes with this means that I can be completely honest with you about my frustrations, within the safety of His embrace and grace. As I share with you some of my own moments of disillusionment and extreme irritation, let me invite you to also be honest with God and yourself about such matters. I encourage you not to deny these feelings; instead, admit them and take them to a loving Father. Tell Him you "just don't get it" and openly and humbly ask Him to help you work through them.

I want to share a few key passages and themes from the Bible that initially seemed so painful but, ironically, the Lord has used to bring great healing to my soul. It is exciting to know the power of the

Scriptures in this way as God opens our eyes to see Him and His Word as He intended, stripping us of our own deductions and teaching us not to rely on our own understanding (Prov. 3:5).

When I initially started to explore what the Bible had to say about infertility, the first thing I did was look up the most obvious couples who had encountered this issue in their lives.

Simple, I thought. *Surely I will just be able to find out how they dealt with it and follow their godly example. Easy.* How mistaken I was!

With each couple I added to my list, my "logical reasoning" turned first to disappointment and then to full-blown resentment. As I jotted down the names of each couple, their particular experience, and outcome, I could no longer constrain my tongue.

"Are you kidding me, Lord?" I exploded. "Is this some sort of cruel joke? How is this supposed to help anybody? In fact, knowing this stuff just makes me feel worse than before I started!"

Indignant, I actually read aloud to God each couple in turn, as if He didn't realize they were in the book He had written.

"Abram and Sarai. Humph! They had a son—Isaac" (Gen. 16:1, 21:5).

"Isaac and Rebekah? Oh, twins boys this time, Jacob and Esau" (Gen. 25:21).

"Jacob and Rachel? O look, Lord, they had Joseph and Benjamin" (Gen. 30:1).

"Mmm, I wonder what happened with Manoah and his wife. Of course," I said sarcastically, "they too had a baby: Samson" (Judg. 13:2–3).

"Well, here we are, at arguably the most famous infertile couple in the Bible, Hannah and Elkannah. Not content with just one son—Samuel—they went on to have three more sons and two daughters!" (1 Sam. 1:1–2:11).

This was getting to be beyond a joke. I hadn't come across one couple so far that hadn't been granted their wish. This wasn't helping me at all! On I went . . .

"The Shunammite woman and her husband? Yep, they had a wee boy too" (2 Kings 4:14–17).

"Elizabeth and Zechariah? Well, we all know their baby was John the Baptist" (Luke 1:5–7).

I was bewildered by what I was reading. I could not relate to a single woman or example to follow. I was in a quandary and confused about where to turn for guidance from someone who actually "got it."

FROM SHAME TO SECURITY

As I searched the Scriptures, at last I found a woman who remained childless the whole of her life. Her name was Michal, daughter of King Saul who became wife to King David (2 Sam. 6). When this girl fell in love with the totally gorgeous David, I'm sure she dreamed theirs would a long, happy, and fruitful marriage. However, as time passed and misunderstandings and betrayal entered their relationship, Michal ended up feeling nothing but disgust and resentment toward her husband.

Their problems came to a head one day as she watched David dancing in the street, half dressed, celebrating the return of the Ark of the Covenant to Jerusalem. This proud girl, more concerned about how David looked in front of his subjects than his worship of God, was mortified at his behavior and, "despised him her heart" (v16b), never held back in telling him so. Exasperated and fed up with her haughtiness and constant attacks on his character, David told her she could stuff her attitude and that he wanted little more to do with her. It's right after this incident that we read "And Michal the daughter of Saul had no child to the day of her death" (v23). The reason she remained barren is most likely because David refused to sleep with her from that day on; nonetheless, some suggest the implication is that her childlessness was a punishment or judgement brought on by her behaviour toward her husband.

As I read through her story again, my mind started to go into overdrive.

Uh oh, I thought. *That's it! Stephan and I are being punished because of previous sins in our lives.*

Now it all made sense. What had I been thinking? Of course this was the most obvious explanation, especially given how reckless and just a little wild I had been in my youth. In no time at all, I had completely convinced myself that our infertility was a result of our past mistakes and a constant reminder of just how far we had gone (individually and together) in our rebellious attitudes and behavior toward God. I started to see how the *disgrace of barrenness* as mentioned in the Bible was linked to the assumption that God used barrenness as a judgement, withholding His blessing from those who had been disobedient or unrepentant. Now I was completely wracked with guilt and shame. I truly believed we were being punished and would bear the weight of this sentence for the rest of our lives.

At this point, you may need to pause for a moment and take a deep breath. Perhaps this is exactly the place you find yourself in now, and your head is spinning with the same kind of thoughts. If so, don't be afraid to admit this to yourself, your spouse, and to God. I can assure you, you are not alone, and God understands.

Over the years I have come across all types of women with the same feelings of guilt, believing they are completely under the judgement of God in this area of their lives. When someone feels judged or punished, it is usually as a result of doing something wrong, i.e. sin; the only question then is, what is the sin that an individual or couple personally associate with being infertile?

Interestingly, while there are any number of sins that can be implicated, I have noticed that women in particular often associate their barrenness with past or present sexual sin and have given reasons ranging from childhood abuse, sex before marriage, promiscuity, adultery, STD's, and even the belief they have married the wrong partner. All of these areas can affect a woman so deeply, leaving her with crippling guilt and shame that seems to smother her consciousness of the love of Christ. It would be impossible to cover all these particular aspects, so I've highlighted only a couple of examples I've heard expressed from questioning, aching hearts over the years that have particularly touched my heart.

The first is to do with the issue of contraception. A recent conversation I had with a young woman is typical of others I have encountered and reflects the thoughts of many women predominantly struggling in the early stages of infertility. For the previous 10 years of her life, this girl had been using a hormone-based contraceptive and now, trying for a baby and being unsuccessful, she had automatically linked her problem conceiving with her years of using this type of contraception. While there is little scientific evidence that prolonged use of hormone-based prophylactics have a detrimental effect on fertility, some anecdotal evidence suggests that around 70-80% of all pregnancies occurring in the first month after a woman has ceased long-term use of a hormonal contraceptive end in early miscarriage. On having suffered her ninth miscarriage, this girl had concluded that since she had artificially manipulated her hormones to induce an unnatural response in her body, she had gone against God's design for her body and was now dealing with the repercussions of her actions. She believed her infertility to be a consequence of her self-indulgent choices, and her difficulties were a direct judgement from God.

This train of thought may seem ridiculous to those who have never experienced problems conceiving, but it is very common among women who are looking to pin the reason for their pain onto something or someone.

The second area in which many women struggle to overcome deep-rooted and intense feelings of guilt is that of having terminated a pregnancy through abortion or having potentially done so by taking the morning-after pill.

"Why would God give me another child when I prevented the life of one He may have gifted me with earlier in my life? Why would He entrust a life to my womb when that was the very place I potentially or definitely ended another's? The safest place that baby should have been became . . . "

Sometimes the response trails off, unable to be answered completely because these are huge questions with profound implications for our lives. When confronted within the context of infertility, these questions can leave a woman drowning in shame, guilt, and hopelessness. These women cannot forgive themselves and therefore find it even more unbelievable to fathom how a Holy God could truly forgive them either. Every single month the reality of their emptiness reinforces their feelings of undeservedness, confirming their belief that they brought this "judgement" on themselves and now, like Michal, will "bear this cross" for the rest of their lives.

But is this true? Does God punish us in this way? Did we really create our own problems and are we reaping what we've sown? This type of shame, brought on for whatever reason, holds many of us in silence, and we dare not voice our dreads and fears. What if our friends and family were to find out the extent of our sins? Would our church be able to handle it? Where do we go with these insecurities and questions that seem to be taking over our rational minds?

I will be forever thankful that God placed a heart of faith in Stephan that never once questioned the nature of the Father's care toward us. He was not even slightly persuaded by my reasoning. No one could convince him that his loving Heavenly Father, who had given everything He had in His Son Jesus in order to take the penalty for our sin, was now going to "crucify Him all over" by punishing us again.

"There's just no way, Jo. God doesn't work that way. That's not who He is, and His character won't let Him."

Stephan then went on to remind me of 1 John 1:9, that says, "If we confess our sins, He is faithful and just to forgive us our sins and to cleanse us from all unrighteousness." He reminded me that *all* means all, and if we confess our sin, there is nothing that is unforgivable and not covered with the blood of Jesus.

You see, girls, when we take a step back and think about it, because of who God is and because He is full of mercy and grace, it does not make sense on any level that God would bring our infertility on us as a judgement.

The problem, though, is that we don't always see it this way because our emotions have become the thing that determines how we perceive our life and God's Word. Marie Durso writes that "feelings are the greatest distorter of revelation. Our emotions oftentimes hide the truth of God's Word. So even though you want to believe what the Bible says, it's as though there is a blockage in the brain of your heart." I would agree with her. If you are struggling to understand God's revelation during this time, then this is one of the junctures in your story where you need to ask the Holy Spirit to help you rightly connect your head/mind with your heart/emotions.

There was a time when I also needed to do this and had to ask God to give me a new understanding of the immensity of His forgiveness, a forgiveness without limit or condition. He taught me all over again what it meant that "There is therefore now no condemnation for those who are in Christ Jesus. For the law of the Spirit of life has set you free in Christ Jesus" (Rom. 8:1-2b).

In those hours and days of feeling judged and broken by guilt, let your heart soak in these words, knowing they were written for you: "For God did not send his Son into the world to condemn the world, but in order that the world might be saved through Him" (John 3:17).

Jesus reminded me that it is completely by grace that I am saved (Eph. 2:8), and had I lived my life any differently, it wouldn't have made one bit of difference to the sacrifice that He would still have had to make to buy me back. I'm not even sure we really get or understand what His grace means, but my favorite definition of grace is "one-way love [from God]." It's Him doing for us what we could never do for ourselves. Isn't that amazing? It has nothing at all to do with us because it's God showing His love to us, whether we receive it or not. He is always going to love us, no matter what we have done or are going to do. He is full of grace (one-way love), mercy, and truth.

Christ will show us when we are believing the lies of the enemy and where we are condemning ourselves for sins He has already paid for. He will encourage us that "for whenever our hearts condemn us, God is greater than our hearts and He knows everything" (1 John 3:20). He is so amazing and has the power, means, and willingness to set us free, if we'd only let Him.

The question is how do we find this out? How to we begin to see for ourselves this incredible person of Jesus and understand His grace? How do we even begin to climb out of this swirling spiral of despair to find freedom and security in Christ?

Can I suggest that you not make your first port of call with a counselor, friend, or even support group? First and foremost, open your Bible. As you read, ask the Holy Spirit to make it a "lamp to your feet and a light to your path" (Psalm 119:105). If there is one thing I would beg you to do, it's to get into reading God's Word because that's how He reveals Himself and shows us the truth. "The unfolding of your words gives light; it imparts understanding to the simple" (Psalm 119:130). It's how He turns our shame into security in Him. When we grasp that and surrender our unbelief, sin, and lives to Him, we will know He is working in us for His good pleasure.

The same Bible that you initially felt condemned you will be the thing that sets you free and gives you inspiration for your future. As God's words set your heart alight with a new vitality and love, you will want to read it more and more. It will become your strength and go-to for your daily dependence and communion with Him. When you do as John Owen said and "feed on His Word, mix it with faith and let it diffuse into our very souls," it will transform you and open your eyes to blessing where there was once only pain.

As I explored the Bible more, I discovered a few other women for whom I think this concept might have been true. These are all women who are suspected to have been childless but nonetheless had a great impact for God and influence on His people in their day. Sometimes I smile at how ironic it is that God took my initial frustration generated by barren women in the Bible and used women of whom there is no mention of children as examples to follow. This is the kind of God we have though, and over and over again in my life, I see how He takes the things that could be the source of much sadness and turns them into the sweetest blessings. Sometimes I think He does this to give us just a little hint of what heaven will be like when He redeems all the bad stuff and shows us how good, perfect, and wonderful everything was originally intended to be.

I've only given you the briefest of summaries of the lives of some of these incredible women of God, but I urge you to spend more time in your own Bible and look them up and be inspired by their lives and testimonies.

OLD TESTAMENT GALS:

Miriam: Big sister to Moses, Miriam was a key influence in the life of this mighty man of God, from the time he was placed in the bulrushes to his leading the children of Israel through the wilderness. This woman was considered a great leader in her own right among God's people—"I sent before you Moses, Aaron, and Miriam" (Micah 6:4b)—and tradition holds that her husband was Hur, a godly man who held up Moses' hands to win the battle (Ex. 17:12). There is no record either in Scripture or in tradition of Miriam's children. It is believed she was childless all her days.

Jehosheba: I love this gal because, like me, she was a doting aunty to her precious little nephew, Joash. When he was born, Joash was actually a threat to the reigning queen, Athaliah, for the right to the throne. This wicked monarch set out to kill Joash and many others. Aunty Jehosheba managed to sneak him out and, as her husband was a priest, they hid him in the temple for seven years. After this time, Jehosheba's husband gathered together the army and brought little Joash out, and they overthrew Athaliah in one day. Although it doesn't seem they had their own kids, their hand in the life of their nephew had a huge positive influence on the whole kingdom of Judah for years to come while Joash reigned (2 Kings 11:1–21, 2 Chron. 22:10–24:1).

Huldah: This woman was a prophetess who lived around the same time as Zephaniah and Jeremiah. She was considered an academic in her time. She was smart and used her intellect to serve and speak for God. Although she does appear to have been married, there is no mention of any children (2 Kings 22–24, 2 Chron. 34).

Esther: Esther was a young Jewish girl who ended up winning a beauty contest to become the queen of the Persian Empire. Faced with what looked like certain death, she went on to save a whole nation from genocide. Quite a girl! But there is no mention at all of Esther being a mother. Imagine if Esther had not been interested or active in anything else in life other than being a mother. If this had been her primary concern, it is possible she might not have been in a position to be used of God in the way that she was. This great opportunity to be involved in the lives of God's people and to grow immensely in her own faith may have passed her by if she had not been who and where she was at that time (Book of Esther).

NEW TESTAMENT GALS:

Anna: The Bible introduces us to this lady when she was about 84 years old. She had been married only seven years before being widowed and went on to live the rest of her life at the temple in Jerusalem. She spent her days and nights there, fasting and praying and worshipping. Her lifestyle alone indicates she was almost certainly childless (Luke 2:36–38). There are women of prayer . . . and then there's Anna!

Joanna: This girl was married to a wealthy, important man who managed King Herod's house. It's probable that she helped support Jesus and His disciples financially. For a time she traveled with Jesus and His band of followers, which would have been an unlikely occurrence if she'd had children at home. After having watched Jesus be crucified, she was one of the girls who went to tend to His dead body, only to be one of this first to discover He had risen (Luke 8:1–3, 23:55–24:12).

The woman with a discharge of blood: This poor woman had bled for twelve years and, being considered "ceremoniously unclean" for that whole time, she would have had to keep her distance from people around her. She would never have known a friend's or lover's tender touch. Her loneliness I can only imagine was a constant agony. When in desperation she reached out to touch Jesus garment and was healed, he said to her, "And he said to her, 'Daughter, your faith has made you well; go in peace'" (Luke 8:48). Just like this trembling woman, if we come to Jesus in faith, believing He is the only one with the power to heal us, then this is where we will find peace for our lives too.

The Samaritan Woman: This lone girl who had lived a colorful life bumped into Jesus one day as she went to collect water from the well. As the two of them got into conversation, there is no mention of children, only her "husbands." Could it have been that her promiscuity was linked to her infertility, that she was looking for a man who could give her a child? Perhaps she had been used and abused by the men in her life because she was unable to bear them children. There is no way to know for sure, but it does seem a little odd that her kids, if she had any, weren't at the well with her. Anyway, after she met Jesus none of that mattered because "many Samaritans from that town believed in Him because of [her] testimony." And when she brought them to meet Jesus, "many more believed because of His Word" (John 4). The testimony of this one woman changed her whole town! Now that's a missionary gal to learn from!

Dorcas: Serving in the coastal port town of Joppa, Dorcas probably helped look after the many widows and fatherless children whose husbands or dads had been lost at sea. There is never any mention of her husband or children, and when she unexpectedly dies, it is Peter who is sent for (Acts 9:36–42).When Peter supernaturally raises her back to life, she just gets up and resumes her service! Now that's a gal with a servant's heart!

Priscilla: She was one half of the dynamic husband and wife duo "Priscilla and Aquila," who risked their lives to serve the church. Dear and trusted friends of Paul, they are held in high regard and mentioned seven times, indicating their influence among God's people. Paul writes, "Not only I, but all the churches of the Gentiles are grateful to them." However, there is no indication that they had any children and no mention given of their children. It may have been that being childless allowed them to work within a particular sphere of risky and time-consuming ministry that they perhaps would have been unable to complete otherwise (Rom. 16:3–4, Acts 18, 1 Cor. 16:19, 2 Tim. 4:19).

Perhaps the most noticeable thing about these women of faith is that they all seem to have a definite purpose to their lives apart from producing and raising children. In different ways and through different experiences, they all had another goal of being faithful to God, following Christ, and serving His people. Some of these girls may have indeed had children, we can't be entirely sure, but regardless, it is not their role or service as a mother that God chooses to record in the Scriptures. They are all recognized because of their devotion to Christ and a life lived in pursuit of His kingdom. Girls, there is more, so much more to our lives than just having a family. The Bible is full of people who were focused on the world to come rather than this one. Let us endeavour to be women and couples like that, who will one day hear "well done, good and faithful servant" because we have done just that—served faithfully. We will have completed the work He had for us to do and not been crippled by shame or frozen by fear because we will have learned to fight our guilt and fear with His Word and allowed Him to work in us (Phil. 2:13).

A PROBLEM WITH PROVERBS

PROVERBS 30:15–16

> *"The leech has two daughters: Give and Give. Three things are never satisfied; four never say, "Enough": Sheol, the barren womb, the land never satisfied with water, and the fire that never says, "Enough."*

For years, these seemed to me to be the craziest, most nonsensical words I had ever read in the whole Bible. Undoubtedly, more than any other reference to infertility in the Scriptures, this is the passage I struggled with most of all: "the barren womb . . . never says enough." In other words, there are some things in life that will never be satisfied, that will cause constant restlessness, and from which no peace can be found—in this case, an unfruitful womb craving for a baby.

For an infertile woman, is this not a cruel verse indeed? Could there be any more crushing words?

Exasperated and frustrated, I had many conversations with God about these verses. And when I say *conversation*, I really mean one-way rants:

"Is that it Lord? Is this all I can look forward to? Is it not distressing enough that I cannot get pregnant, but now you're telling me that on top of that, these burning desires will never ease, never be resolved?"

If this interpretation was indeed true, then it was a conundrum to me how any barren woman could continue to live and have any peace in her life. Ultimately, it would be too much to bear. This Scripture was crushing to my spirit, and the result was that I became angry and resentful and so decided for the most part to just try and ignore it.

Problem was, no matter how much I tried to forget these words, I couldn't. On top of that, the irresponsible mishandling of this text by a number of Bible teachers—whether written or spoken—only reinforced my feelings of complete despair and resignation. As I read various commentaries or sat under teachings on barrenness, sometimes I would bristle inside with indignation toward the teacher and think, *how dare you presume to speak on such matters in such a flippant and matter-of-fact way when you have absolutely no idea of the impact this has on people's lives!*

This examination of the way others interpreted Proverbs 30 (and other passages to do with infertility) only compounded my feelings of confusion and sadness and strengthened my resolve to ignore this part of God's Word. I blamed those so-called scholars for my confusion and used them to justify the attitude of my heart and validate my "righteous anger" toward not only them but ultimately God Himself. This was my excuse anyway. In truth, I was probably more afraid than ever of these verses and the implications they may have for my life.

As with so much in my life, God patiently waited for me and eventually brought me to a place of repentance and safety. Eventually I asked him, "Lord, help me to understand these words. I don't know what they mean, and they seem to conflict with what I already know about you and your character. But, they are written for a reason, and I want to accept the whole truth of your Word."

FROM FRUSTRATION TO FREEDOM

As I prayed and asked God to help me to understand, the Holy Spirit began to show me things in a new light. What He revealed to me, I never found in any commentary nor heard from any platform. It was not eloquent or complicated but nonetheless deeply affected my soul. In essence, I began to have a fresh understanding of the true heart and character of God the Father and my identity in and standing before Him.

The Holy Spirit reminded me that God is not only my perfect Father, referring to how I should see Him, but I am also His daughter, referring to how He sees me. Okay, you may say, nothing new or startling there. We know that we are born again into God's family and that we are His children; it's the same for every Christian. Sometimes though, I think as Christians we hear these truths so often that we can become desensitized to the implications of them. Just take a few minutes and ponder this fact for a moment: We have been adopted into the family of God and are joint heirs with Jesus!

He reminded me then just how precious I actually am to Him. As someone once said, "the value of something is only determined by how much someone is willing to pay for it." Well, God paid the highest price he could've ever paid to make you and me His own. If we are so precious to Him, does it then make sense that He would leave us with no hope as these verses would suggest? Of course not!

In Christ we are a new creation, and that means that while we do have a new identity and standing before God, He also changes our deepest "unquenchable" desires, hungers, and longings by His power. As He led me gently through these verses, He showed me that for the believer, not only is the never-ending ache of the barren womb a lie but also that none of the four insatiable things mentioned need be true. For each of the four negatives, He gave me positives so much greater and full of promise. I want to focus on the barren womb and share with you how God really did give me beauty for ashes and swapped my mourning for joy.

First, I have a confession to make. I hate that word *barren*. It means to remain fruitless and just sounds so ugly and final. What I dislike most about it in this particular passage is that this connotation of finality forces us to ask how we truly feel at the prospect of *never* being able to bear children of our own. Now that's a question some of us don't even want to think about, but it is often the answer to this very question that will determine how we respond to our desire for a child. These responses generally take one of two forms and can switch at different stages along our journey, depending on our particular circumstances and how long we have been on this road. The first reaction is that of passionate desperation, while the other tends to be more indicative of a reconciled acceptance. Stephan and I as a couple have encountered both emotions along the way.

I remember feeling this first type of response one particular Sunday morning in church. Near the beginning of his sermon, the pastor mentioned this verse in Proverbs 30 as a passing comment of an example of something a woman would always long for and never be rid of for the whole duration of her life. I sat there for the next hour, feeling like I'd been emotionally punched yet again. The rest of the sermon was lost to me. In the days following as I pondered this verse more and more, I thought this must indeed be true, especially when I thought of all the other stories I'd heard about women in their relentless pursuit of fulfilling this ache in them. I've witnessed it over and over again, this yearning, peculiar to the need to carry a child in your womb. So strong is the desire to fill this void that people will go to great lengths in their endeavour to satisfy their emptiness.

When you are in this place and feel the ferocity of this burning desire, it is not difficult to imagine that you will experience these wants for as long as you live. It was when I believed this to be true that my heart, broken with hurt and confusion, began to harden somewhat toward God and His Word. I just could not reconcile in my spirit how a loving Father would inflict this type of pain without providing any way out or any healing for the wounds it appeared He had caused. The strength of such feelings can easily pull you down into a state of complete hopelessness. I was also profoundly confused because even though I thought these words could be true, my reasoning did not seem to match up with what I already knew and had previously experienced of the merciful character of God. Something was definitely wrong with my understanding; I just didn't know what and couldn't seem to find any resolution. And so I stayed in that place of disillusion for way too long.

As time passed however, the intensity of these emotions, powerful as they had been, seemed to settle somewhat. Many couples do indeed find that time makes things easier, and so for them the answer to the question of whether the ache for a child ever subsides may be seasoned with a level of acceptance that would not have been possible a few years earlier.

Finding herself in this season, my friend Ellie told me that after many years of her desires remaining unfulfilled and her prayers seemingly unanswered, she had come to a place of quiet acceptance that motherhood was never going to happen to her and had resigned herself not only to accept her situation but also to believe that it was okay. Her attitude was one of "it's obvious the Lord doesn't want this for me, and so I just have to accept His will and just live with it and deal with it as best I can. No point moping around or allowing this to stop me from living my life with at least some degree of happiness. At the same time, Lord, should You ever change Your mind, I'm definitely up for that, but for now, I guess I just gotta deal."

Nothing wrong with that, you may say. In fact, that sounds like a healthy frame of mind to be in—to have arrived at a place in your life where you have found some resolution to your circumstances and seem to be coping well with your pain. I would wholeheartedly agree that it's good to be able to be free from the intensity of your situation and its damaging effects, especially since some are never able to reach that point. But my Christian brothers and sisters, having gone through times of both intense dissatisfaction and calm resolve, I want to challenge both these views to life.

You see, unbelievers can also eventually achieve some semblance of peace and acceptance in their painful circumstances, but as His children, is this really what God wants for us? Is His plan really for us to now live in a state of benign resignation? I would venture that nothing could be further from the truth! When we consider this word *barren* and its implications for our lives, it doesn't matter if it evokes feelings of intense frustration and anger against God or a calm, collected resignation, if an unquenchable emptiness still lies deep within our souls.

Early one morning while I was out walking with the Lord across the fields, He challenged my heart about this. The reason we find ourselves in a place of quiet acceptance and "manageable" discontentment is because we have reached a point in our lives when we are able to stop asking the *why me* questions about our lack of children. This is what had happened to my friend Ellie. She stopped asking God *"why has this happened to us,"* because she had unknowingly lulled herself into a state of resolution that she felt she could live with and that allowed her to function as normally as possible. Many do this. We get over the intensity of emotions we once had. We know the bitter questions are pointless now. We could live in this state of functional satisfaction for the rest of their lives. But this is a dangerous place for a Christian to remain. As the years pass, this location can become like a miry bog, leaving you stuck in resentment and bitterness, rendered useless for building God's kingdom.

We get stuck not because we stop asking the negative "why me" questions but because we never ask the "why me" questions about the blessings we've received from God. The significance and impact of this truth has the power to change the whole future of any struggling individual or couple.

Let me tell you, when you start to focus on the blessings, He will open your eyes to see and understand just how much you have been flooded by His mercy and grace. These things will thrill your heart more than anything this world offers. Gratitude will overcome your very soul, so that all the things you thought yourself deprived of fade into the background and become almost irrelevant. As your questions change from the sad "why me" to wondering "who am I that you'd even think of me," your heart and your life will transform into the thing of worship that He so wants it to be!

You will be so stirred in your spirit that, rather than living a life of quiet resignation, you'll be unable to keep from praising your Heavenly Father. Your life will no longer be about learning to accept what He hasn't given you. Instead, you will be bursting with joy and wonder at the amazing things He has given you! Your faith will change from a coping strategy to a shining testimony of love and service that comes from a heart that sees and understands just how good our God is. He doesn't want us to find some sort of resolution just so we can become partially contented, happy but "ineffective" childless Christian couples who survive but do nothing for the kingdom. Are you kidding? There is something so much greater than just building a family here on this earth. We have the opportunity to be part of adding to God's family and building up His kingdom. God has placed you where He has with the intention that we live our lives to the full, doing what He would have us do, which is no less important because there is an absence of children.

The Holy Spirit gently began to show me that while Christ may not require me to be fruitful in a natural sense, He was definitely guiding me to be involved in making disciples—in other words, to be fruitful in a spiritual sense. At one stage in my life, I would never have believed that I would rather be a "spiritual" mother than a natural one, but God has given me a desire to have "sons and daughters" in the faith that is stronger than my desire for natural children ever was.

I know what you're thinking, "that's just not natural," and you would be right; it's not natural, it's supernatural!

One day not so long ago, a friend asked me if I found it difficult to be present whenever a new baby was being dedicated to the Lord in our church.

"Those mornings must be so hard for you," she sympathized. "How do you manage to get through them when you see everyone celebrating a new baby and there you are, knowing that you'll probably never have one of your own? Is that not the most difficult thing to sit through?" she asked.

I couldn't help but smile to myself as I thought how only that previous week I had been in that exact situation. As I sat and watched the pastor hold this tiny baby boy in his arms and pray over him and his parents, I felt a slight thrill well up in my own heart. As he asked God to help this little one's parents raise him well and that one day this child too would make the choice to follow Jesus, I was blown away yet again by some of the amazing opportunities God has granted me. You see, what this pastor gets to do for this infant on a Sunday morning, I get to do on a Monday morning!

During the course of my everyday life, I have some level of interaction with young single moms and teenage mothers. Their kids aren't likely to be taken to the front of a church to be prayed over, they're not likely to be raised by parents who love Jesus, not likely to have a church family to help steer them in the right paths throughout their lives. No, these are babies whose first words will probably include swear words because that's what they hear most often. Our kids in Sunday school love to sing, "we're God's amazing children," and so they are, but when I listen to them, God reminds me that so are those little babies and young children I see every week who may never attend Sunday school.

That particular Sunday as I watched the pastor hold that baby boy, I thought of the little girl I'd held in my arms just a couple of days earlier. She was only seven months old, freezing with no socks and no coat. Her mother was calling her every name under the sun, swearing because the baby hadn't slept well during the night and mommy was hung over from partying the night before.

"Okay, Lord," I muttered in my mind, "this is not cool on any level; this doesn't seem fair, whichever way you cut it."

As quickly as those thoughts entered my head, the Holy Spirit answered right back, "Don't go there, Jo, don't forget what I've taught you. This is an opportunity to love on this wee one, so don't waste it."

In those moments, though not in front of a congregation, I get to hold that little one and look into her eyes and commit her wee life to Christ, praying for His protection over her and the salvation of her soul. I get to pray for her mother, and encourage and love on her mother for that short time.

Or it could be a day when another teenage girl excitedly runs up to me. "Jo, I'm pregnant!"

"Yeah, and you're seventeen, and your life's a mess, and this time next month your baby daddy is probably gonna be in prison or have left you for someone else," comes my initial unspoken retort. But then I get to pray for her and her unborn child. I get to help her with her physical needs and lift her spirit on her bad days. With every ultrasound picture she brings me, I see the hand of sin and am reminded that where sin abounds, grace abounds all the more (Rom 5:20) and that God can redeem even this situation.

Or maybe it's a day when a young teenage father, involved in sectarian gang life and dabbling in the occult, comes to my door with his two-week-old son. "Jo, I've brought the wee man down to see you—you want to hold him?" As he tells me how precious this little one is to him, I am afforded the privilege of encouraging this young man and praying silently over his new son, for God's protection over his wee life and that one day both him and his father will be led to Christ and both be amazing men of God.

You see, I live with the hope and the dream that someday, I am going to meet some of these babies and their moms or dads in heaven when they will come up to me and say, "I'm here, in part, because you prayed that God would bring someone into my life to lead me to Jesus and He did," or "Jo, I met Jesus because, in part, you showed me His grace and loved me when no one else did." Or "Jo, I had a life because you talked my mother out of having an abortion."

Guys, this is the stuff I live for; the very fact that I might have the privilege to perhaps be involved in someone's journey of salvation is what gets me up in the mornings, no matter who it is. In these instances, these kids come to me, not because I can give them the best pregnancy tips or parenting advice, but for the grace that Jesus has shown toward us. When you share that grace with others, the Holy Spirit will keep pouring it into you so that it blesses and transforms you in ways that words can't express. You will truly know that not only is His grace sufficient for you (Eph. 2:8), but it's also sufficient for them.

So am I sitting in the pew on a Sunday morning, pouting, wishing that was us and our baby? Are you kidding me? Sometimes I want to jump up from my seat because my heart is bursting with the wonder of being able to pray not just for that baby but so many others. It's no longer about what seems fair in our eyes but about the honour and privilege of being a link in someone else's journey into the family of God.

While I realize I have taken this verse somewhat out of context, nonetheless, these words can be true for those of us in whom God has placed the desire to be a spiritual mother:

"Sing, O barren one, who did not bear;

Break forth into singing and cry aloud,

You who have not been in labour!

For the children of the desolate one will be more

than the children of her who is married," says the Lord.

- Isaiah 54:1

But, girls, I was most definitely not always in that place. It took years before Jesus brought that change about in my life. So please don't expect to walk into church on Mother's Day full of the joys of spring while you are still walking through the tender parts of your journey. But as you go along, take courage, and as you step out gingerly in faith, ask Christ to help you with this particular area, and He will. He will supernaturally turn your mourning into joy. How He will do it in your life, I do not know. I'm sure it'll be very different from anyone else's experience, but however He chooses, He will become a balm for your aching heart.

He takes us beyond what the world accepts as a good and healthy state of mind to a place of complete freedom that will make your heart sing even in these potentially heart-wrenching situations. When Christ gets a hold of you—and if we allow it—He can satisfy those yearnings that you might now believe are forever unquenchable and place in your heart an even stronger desire for Him and the plans He has for your life.

He will do this as you read His Word. I'm sure half my friends want to run away when they see me because they know I'm going to ask them if they are reading their Bible. Friends, I cannot even begin to put into words how vital it is for your spiritual growth during this season of your life to read His Word every day. The Scriptures will raise you from being in a relationship with Christ to being in *fellowship* with Him. It's that which will sustain you in your weakest moments.

Be encouraged by the words of George Muller, that wonderful man of prayer who devoted his life building orphanages for the 'lost' children of Bristol, who said:

> The power of our spiritual life will be according to the measure of the room that the Word of God takes up in our life and in our thoughts. After an experience of fifty-four years, I can solemnly declare this. For three years after my conversion I used the Word little. Since that time I searched it with diligence, and the blessing was wonderful. From that time, I have read the Bible through a hundred times in order, and at every time with increasing joy. Whenever I start freshly with it, it appears to me as a new book. I cannot express how great the blessing is of faithful, daily, regular searching of the Bible. The day is lost for me, on which I have used no rounded time for enjoying the Word of God.

CHAPTER 4

OUR CHILD SACRIFICE

IT WAS A BEAUTIFUL, SUNNY morning. With the kids away at school and Stephan gone for work, I planned to get busy with some spring cleaning. Housework, I confess, is not one of my natural talents, and by the time I was vacuuming the third bedroom, I was thoroughly fed up. Taking a break from the cleaning, I snuggled down—as was my habit—into a little recessed window in my bedroom to spend a little time reading the Bible. This particular morning, I was drawn for no peculiar reason to read the story of Abraham in Genesis 22. I didn't even make it past the first verse of the passage when I was floored.

It was one of those times when the power of God's Word hit me with such a force that I felt like I could not speak or even breathe properly. I was riveted to that window seat and couldn't have moved even if I'd wanted to. His presence was so enveloping that I wanted to stay there forever as He began to reveal to me from this story some answers to some of my feelings of frustration concerning our infertility.

Just take a few minutes and read the story of Abraham taking his son Isaac up the mountain to offer him as a sacrifice to God (Genesis 22:1–19).

> **1** After these things God tested Abraham and said to him, "Abraham!" And he said, "Here I am." **2** He said, "Take your son, your only son Isaac, whom you love, and go to the land of Moriah, and offer him there as a burnt offering on one of the mountains of which I shall tell you." **3** So Abraham rose early in the morning, saddled his donkey, and took two of his young men with him, and his son Isaac. And he cut the wood for the burnt offering and arose and went to the place of

which God had told him. *4* On the third day Abraham lifted up his eyes and saw the place from afar. *5* Then Abraham said to his young men, "Stay here with the donkey; I and the boy will go over there and worship and come again to you." *6* And Abraham took the wood of the burnt offering and laid it on Isaac his son. And he took in his hand the fire and the knife. So they went both of them together. *7* And Isaac said to his father Abraham, "My father!" And he said, "Here I am, my son." He said, "Behold, the fire and the wood, but where is the lamb for a burnt offering?" *8* Abraham said, "God will provide for himself the lamb for a burnt offering, my son." So they went both of them together. *9* When they came to the place of which God had told him, Abraham built the altar there and laid the wood in order and bound Isaac his son and laid him on the altar, on top of the wood. *10* Then Abraham reached out his hand and took the knife to slaughter his son. *11* But the angel of the Lord called to him from heaven and said, "Abraham, Abraham!" And he said, "Here I am." *12* He said, "Do not lay your hand on the boy or do anything to him, for now I know that you fear God, seeing you have not withheld your son, your only son, from me." *13* And Abraham lifted up his eyes and looked, and behold, behind him was a ram, caught in a thicket by his horns. And Abraham went and took the ram and offered it up as a burnt offering instead of his son. *14* So Abraham called the name of that place, "The Lord will provide", as it is said to this day, "On the mount of the Lord it shall be provided."

15 And the angel of the Lord called to Abraham a second time from heaven *16* and said, "By myself I have sworn, declares the Lord, because you have done this and have not withheld your son, your only son, *17* I will surely bless you, and I will surely multiply your offspring as the stars of heaven and as the sand that is on the seashore. And your offspring shall possess the gate of his enemies, **18** and in your offspring shall all the nations of the earth be blessed, because you have obeyed my voice." **19** So Abraham returned to his young men, and they arose and went together to Beersheba. And Abraham lived at Beersheba.

As a little girl in Sunday school, I thought this story was nothing short of horrific. To be honest, I never really understood it.

"Why would a caring God ask this of any parent?" I would ask myself.

The whole thing seemed completely unreasonable, if not cruel. Over time, though, the Holy Spirit taught me to see this story through different eyes, to see what I thought was completely "nuts" as so sweet and encouraging. Indeed, probably more than any other, this is the Scripture that softened my heart and revolutionized how I view the role of infertility in my life.

While I am eager to share my gleanings with you, don't let what I write be the limit of your thoughts. This is God's Word, not mine, and therein lies the power. Before we go any further, take a moment to pray and ask the Holy Spirit to help you surrender your mind to Him. Perhaps read the story again, slowly this time, and allow God's Word to wash over you.

Abraham's Silence (vs 1-2): "**1** After these things God tested Abraham and said to him, "Abraham!" And he said, "Here I am." **2** He said, "Take your son, your only son Isaac, whom you love, and go to the land of Moriah, and offer him there as a burnt offering on one of the mountains of which I shall tell you."

Almost immediately, I was struck by how one sided this conversation seemed between Abraham and God. It appears God was doing all the talking. Abraham remained quiet as God told him plainly what he was to do with Isaac. There was no debating between the two of them, no question of whether Abraham would agree or any consideration given to what he might feel the limits of his sacrifice should be.

I have to admit, I found this a little strange and somewhat out of character for Abraham. Remember, this is a guy who had quite a gutsy personality, boldly bartering with God to spare Sodom for his nephew Lot.

Another time, upon hearing Lot had been captured, Abraham immediately rallied all his fighting men and went after the kidnappers in the middle of the night. He not only rescued his relatives and recovered all their stolen possessions, but he also drove out the whole army of captors.

Furthermore, not long before this particular incident with Isaac, God had told Abraham he must also give up his other son, Ishmael. In that instance, Abraham immediately made it known that "the thing was very displeasing to [him] on account of his son" (Gen. 21:11). There is no doubt Abraham was a passionate guy who didn't leave people wondering what he thought about a situation.

So why now all of a sudden does he seem so passive and resigned to God's request? I suspect there is something else that Abraham had discovered over the course of his life as he grew in friendship with God.

I think Abraham had come to realize that ultimately God is the one who chooses our sacrifices—we don't get to pick our own!

This idea blew me away. As I pondered it more, it occurred to me that infertility may indeed be the sacrifice God was asking of us. I began to see more clearly that, as in Abraham's situation, it is *God's* choice what He will ask of me in this life, not mine.

I imagine God asks particular things of us because He knows we wouldn't choose these sacrifices for ourselves. I would never have chosen infertility for myself. Let's face it, if it was left up to us to decide on our own crosses to take up daily, they would not likely be heavy or particularly effective for strengthening our faith. So perhaps God selects them for us because He knows we wouldn't or couldn't. We don't always know what's best for us, whereas He does—and that's precisely why He gets to choose!

However, what God allows in one person's life is often completely different in another's. We may not be asked to go through the same hardships that others face, but this particular "infertility sacrifice" could be what God has asked of me. The question now is . . . will I respond like Abraham?

No! . . . well, definitely not in the beginning, anyway. In fact, my response was completely the opposite. Exasperated, I threw myself into questioning and arguing with God.

"Why me? What have I done to deserve this? How can this be fair? I just don't get it, Lord!"

I imagine there have been many times you've responded the same way. Maybe Abraham had similar thoughts in his head, but I think overall his trust in God outweighed his queries and questions. Experience had taught him that His ways are not our ways and His thoughts are not our thoughts (Isaiah 55:8). When we surrender our will to His and resolve to develop a deep friendship with God, we learn, like Abraham, to trust His judgement and change the nature of our questions. Although many of us are not able to offer this sacrifice in a practical way because our infertility is not a choice we can make or decide if we will choose to submit to or not, the stance of our heart can still be sacrificial in how we approach our barrenness.

So, without uttering a word, Abraham rose early the next morning and set off to fulfil God's request.

Abraham's Servants (vs 3–5: 3) So Abraham rose early in the morning, saddled his donkey, and took two of his young men with him, and his son Isaac. And he cut the wood for the burnt offering and arose and went to the place of which God had told him. **4** On the third day Abraham lifted up his eyes and saw the place from afar. **5** Then Abraham said to his young men, "Stay here with the donkey; I and the boy will go over there and worship and come again to you."

Knowing the journey ahead was going to be long and arduous, Abraham took along two helpers. However, as they neared their destination, he turned to his servants and told them they must wait behind. They could only go so far on the journey with Abraham because it was his sacrifice to make and not theirs.

This, ladies, is also often the case with us. Infertility is our particular sacrifice to give. While friends, counselors, and even medical professionals can help us some of the way, they cannot fully appreciate or feel the full import of what we will give up in this life. Be very thankful for friends who will share the weight of your burden along the way, but know there will come a time when we must go that last part of the journey alone, when we realize that despite our incredible support, the reality is principally ours. This is not altogether a bad thing because as we take responsibility for carrying our own load (Gal. 6:5), God will use this part of the journey to develop our walk with Him, to teach us to depend fully on Him as He strengthens us in our faith.

I have a feeling that final leg up the mountain was a very lonely one for Abraham. So many thoughts must have rushed through his head. Being unable to share them with Isaac must have been torture. It is in those quiet moments when we walk alone, when our friends have been left behind, that we feel the full weight of the burden and realize again that ours is a child sacrifice.

I often wonder if, as he looked up and saw the place where he was to sacrifice his son, Abraham thought, "For your glory, Lord, yes maybe . . . but for my good? Of that, I'm not so sure." Although Abraham may have harbored such feelings, he also knew enough of God's true character to know that he had no other option but to trust Him and trust that the end would most definitely result in his good and God's glory. I'm sure he had no idea how this would happen, and I suspect he disagreed with the whole process, but nonetheless he resolved to surrender his will—and his son—to God.

Perhaps you feel much the same and don't understand why God has chosen you to go through this trial. Surely you could honour Him just as well in another way. To be honest, I don't know why either. I think there are some questions that will never be answered until we get to heaven, but I have to trust that He knows more than I do. Looking at the whole of my life from a bird's eye view, God sees the whole picture and not just this season. His plans for us were laid out before we were born, and as He continues to form us, we must learn to trust Him for this time and surrender our dreams, emotions, minds, and bodies to His care.

Abraham's Sacrifice (vs 6-12: 6) And Abraham took the wood of the burnt offering and laid it on Isaac his son. And he took in his hand the fire and the knife. So they went both of them together. *7* And Isaac said to his father Abraham, "My father!" And he said, "Here I am, my son." He said, "Behold, the fire and the wood, but where is the lamb for a burnt offering?" *8* Abraham said, "God will provide for himself the lamb for a burnt offering, my son." So they went both of them together.

9 When they came to the place of which God had told him, Abraham built the altar there and laid the wood in order and bound Isaac his son and laid him on the altar, on top of the wood. *10* Then Abraham reached out his hand and took the knife to slaughter his son. *11* But the angel of the Lord called to him from heaven and said, "Abraham, Abraham!" And he said, "Here I am." *12* He said, "Do not lay your hand on the boy or do anything to him, for now I know that you fear God, seeing you have not withheld your son, your only son, from me."

How did Abraham manage to build the altar without breaking down emotionally? How was he able to bind up Isaac without completely losing his mind? I wonder if at any point he thought about changing his mind. After all, he wasn't sacrificing Isaac for the "good of the great." This was just between him and God, so was it really necessary? Would it really be that bad if he didn't go through with it? On the other hand, maybe he thought, God has already promised me that Isaac is going to carry on my line and will be the father of a great nation, so unless He lied, this will all come to good, I'm sure.

Could it have been that Abraham was remembering when God told him to send his elder son Ishmael out into the desert? (Gen 21:8–21) He knew that by abandoning a young child and his mother in a desert with no shelter, little bread, and one skin of water, they would have virtually no chance of survival. On a natural level, this would have been a death sentence. But God had said He would make a nation of Ishmael, so Abraham had to trust that his son would be supernaturally protected. Did he ever wonder if they made it out of the desert alive, or is this a time when he fully trusted God's promise for Ishmael and, having been through that, had reassurance that God could do the same with Isaac?

The Bible doesn't tell us what was in Abraham's mind. It may have been that by this stage in his life, Abraham's faith in God's promises was so experientially real that when God asked for Isaac, he wasn't going to argue, no matter what he thought.

Regardless of what was going on in his head, the fact remained that Abraham still had to climb the mountain and build the altar. In other words, while he acknowledged God's sovereignty in his mind, it was only after he physically went through the trial that the angel of the Lord said, "now I know that you fear God, seeing you have not withheld your son."

I am convinced one of the most difficult aspects of being a Christian with infertility is allowing what we believe in our minds to dictate our behavior. What Abraham believed about God became evident in his actions. It's so easy for us to say we fully trust God's plan for us, but what evidence is there for that statement? If we really accept that God allows our infertility, how does this sacrifice change our lives practically? The very practical choices that we will make during this journey can have huge implications for the rest of our lives. We may be asked to make decisions that quite literally involve matters of life and death. These are questions that most of our friends will never encounter or even need to think about. The impact of our behavior in this season can have far-reaching effects and has the potential to be a powerful testimony to those around us and a very visible demonstration of our love for God. We'll discuss these issues in more depth later, but for now, as we observe Abraham's actions, the one obvious resulting behavior is that of worship.

> ***Abraham's Worship (vs 13–14)***: **13** And Abraham lifted up his eyes and looked, and behold, behind him was a ram, caught in a thicket by his horns. And Abraham went and took the ram and offered it up as a burnt offering instead of his son. **14** So Abraham called the name of that place, "The Lord will provide", as it is said to this day, "On the mount of the Lord it shall be provided."

When Abraham realized that God was going to spare Isaac's life, his heart was turned to thankfulness, gratitude, and worship. God doesn't order Abraham to go ahead and make another sacrifice. It is Abraham who upon seeing the ram decides to offer it as an act of worship to God.

"Once worship is experienced and understood, that becomes a sacred ground from which all other decisions are made."

~ Ravi Zacharias

This story reminds us potently of God's ultimate replacement sacrifice for us. God took His very best offering and put it on the altar for us when Jesus took our place on the cross. When we truly understand what we were saved from and see who took our place, our hearts should respond in true worship to Jesus. It is only at the cross that we begin to understand the depth of God's loves for us.

Knowing how deep God's love for us runs means we can fully trust Him with our lives, never doubting that He loves us and alone is worthy of our worship. Take some time and just let this knowledge sink into your soul as if for the first time and then see if the questions you were once asking have changed. After what He gave for us, is there really anything He could ask of us that we would not be willing to put on the altar for Him? Trusting in Him brings a whole new perspective to life. Instead of being frustrated, we can find comfort and see it as a privilege to offer willingly what He has asked.

When someone asked the late, great American tennis player, Arthur Ashe, who contracted HIV from a blood transfusion during heart by-pass surgery, why he was not bitter or self-pitying when he was ill through no fault of his own, he responded, "If I were to say 'God, why me?' about the bad things, then I should have said, 'God, why me?' about the good things that happened in my life." We so easily blame God for all the hard times but never seem to give Him credit for all the good stuff.

I was not just a little convicted by this man's story and longed to have a heart like his for my situation. Through time, if we ask Him, God will indeed do this in us and give us a heart of worship that wants to respond to Him. He changes our hearts to no longer ask "why me" questions. Instead of our emotions and minds constantly questioning and blaming Him for our heartache and emptiness, our spirits will be overtaken in worship toward Him. Our focus becomes thanking and praising Him for all the other amazing things He has given us. We stop asking "why would You deny me?" and start asking "who am I that You would bless me so much?"

"Who am I that You have chosen me to be saved? Who am I that You give me breath in my body today? Who am I, that I get to spend all of eternity with Jesus, only because You choose to bless me?"

These are questions I ask myself often, and I'm still blown away by the grace of God to have even thought of me and wonder sometimes why I would even need to ask for anything else. Just take some time, allow yourself some silent moments in His presence, and let your heart begin to appreciate anew how He has blessed you in measures and ways we cannot comprehend. This doesn't mean that we won't still experience heartache, since of course we will, but our grumbling and pouting will turn into joy. We will be the people of whom God says, "the people whom I formed for myself that they might declare my praise" (Isaiah 43:21).

The next time you are sitting in church and hear the pastor say of this passage, "Parents, try placing yourself in Abraham's shoes to understand what agonies he went through," just think to yourself, *I may be childless, but I know what it is to walk that path of child sacrifice every day and understand so well how Jesus takes this pain and turns my heart to worship!*

Life goes on! While this experience was certainly a defining moment for Abraham, it didn't completely dictate the rest of his life. Verse 19 says, "So Abraham returned to his young men, and they arose and went together to Beersheba. And Abraham lived at Beersheba."

How amazing is that! After he'd nearly killed his treasured son, it seems he just went home and lived his life! This incident was not the beginning or the end of God's plans for Abraham. There were still things for him to do in his ordinary, everyday life. He would never forget the pain of that trial, but the experience would by no means stop him from living.

This is so important for us to remember: life does go on. Throughout this journey, we will also feel the aches of the "mountain hike," but when all is said and done, God does not intend the experience of infertility to define us as women. These experiences will change us forever and contribute to who we are, but God has plans for us in our everyday lives too. We must understand that infertility is only a part of who we are. God will use that in us to draw us closer to Him so that we can be confident that our identity is in Jesus. We must recognize that there is much we can do to serve Him in our everyday lives beyond "the sacrifice." Sacrifice is not the only means of demonstrating our worship, so let's not get stuck on the "sacrificial mountain" but go down and live in the place He has put us, enjoy the blessings of everyday life, and fulfil all the other plans He has for us.

Indeed, recently a friend told me that while she didn't necessarily view her infertility as a sacrifice, she did see it as a God-given opportunity to introduce other precious blessings in her life. She said that had she borne her own natural children, it is likely that she would never have become a foster and adoptive parent and had the amazing blessing and privilege of raising her two wonderful adopted children. She went on to say that for her, infertility was part of God's plan to turn her thoughts to helping parentless babies. It was not necessarily that she had been "denied" childbirth and left with a painful yearning, but instead her barrenness was a route through which others could be blessed. How wonderfully inspiring this woman is!

Whether God has children planned for your future or not, make one outcome of your fertility sure in that, as you walk this path, you will have grown in your friendship with God and have cultivated a relationship with Jesus that is more precious and valuable than anything you could ever have hoped for. How exciting is that! And one day when we meet Him face to face, we will know that it was all worth it and understand then why "our sacrifice is not of our choosing."

CHAPTER 5

GIVE UP YOUR HOPE

YOU MIGHT THINK IT A little strange to be encouraged to give up your hope. Sounds bizarre, but this was among the earliest and most powerful lessons Christ taught me during my journey. It is my prayer that you too will have the courage to re-examine where and in whom your hope is truly placed, specifically for this season of infertility.

Do comments made by well-intentioned friends, like "don't give up hope . . . you never know what might happen," leave you feeling less hopeful than you felt before? Such remarks, borne out of awkwardness and cloaked as encouragement, rarely lift us up as we live through the same cycle of hope turning to despair month after month. Holding onto our hope is exhausting.

Statements meant to encourage me instead elicited a negative response in my heart, and I finally realized why. It was because I didn't have a true understanding of what hope actually meant, and my hope had been completely misplaced. As I looked at the way the Bible talks about hope, I began to see my need of a real hope with a foundation of assurance and certainty. Applying the wrong hope to my life would only lead to disillusionment, disappointment, and sorrow.

The word *hope* is usually used to convey a feeling of expectation that something good will happen sometime in the future; it carries with it a sense of chance or probability. This can often be in the context of referring to things that are somewhat inconsequential in order to indicate our particular preference; for example, "I hope they win the game," or "I hope it doesn't rain today." Many times when people say "stay hopeful," they actually mean "stay upbeat or optimistic." That is, in part, why you can be left feeling empty if not a little confused.

On the other hand, there's a type of hope that doesn't denote our superficial preferences but focuses on the deep longings and strong desires of our hearts. When we think of hope in this way, it means we're placing our trust in something or someone in order to fulfil a yearning within us. We give ourselves over to the power of that circumstance, person, or thing to provide us with the satisfaction, safety, and completeness we seek. We believe that if we trust in those things, then they will take care of us and fulfil an emptiness in our lives.

The Bible is full of verses and passages about hope, and while it's not my intention to present a Bible study on hope, I want to share just a few key passages that have become key anchors in my testimony.

The first is 1 Peter 1:3–4:

> *Blessed be the God and Father of our Lord Jesus Christ!*
>
> *According to his great mercy, he has caused us to be born again*
>
> *to a living hope through the resurrection of Jesus Christ from the dead,*
>
> *to an inheritance that is imperishable, undefiled, and unfading,*
>
> *that is kept in heaven for you.*

Perhaps you have read this verse many times without feeling its impact on your soul. That was my experience until one particular day while reading, I was completely blown away by its truth, as if seeing for the first time what it meant for Christ and the promise of our heavenly inheritance to be my "living hope." I admit, up until then I had not grasped the reality that our hope had to be in, through, and from Christ. Maybe I had viewed Him as the one to fulfil our hopes (of having a baby) but not as the focus or center of our hope. He taught me that absolutely everything and everyone in this world has the potential to die, disappear, or be taken away from us and therefore, if we placed our hope in any of these things and then lost them, our hope would be lost too. The question for us as childless couples then, is if our hope is centered on having a baby and it doesn't happen, do we then have no hope? God forbid!

I have noticed in younger Christian women, especially among those in the early stages of their infertility journey, a real sense of prevailing hope and belief that they will still yet become mothers. Much of their communication would indicate they have never even considered the possibility that this may never happen for them. All their hope is placed in the prospect of becoming pregnant and having a child. At first, I wasn't sure why this bothered me so much. After all, isn't it a good thing to be positive? If you lose hope, you lose everything, right? While I would agree with that in part, the reason I felt unsettled and concerned was because the crucial matter with regards to these women was where they placed their hope. This is hugely important because I truly believe that as we continue further down the path of infertility, so much of the heartache, disappointment, and anger we experience is borne out of misplaced hope.

I remember my aunt telling me of a friend of hers who lived her whole life hanging on to the hope that she would one day have a baby of her own. From the very outset of her married life, all this girl wanted was to be a mommy. However, suffering endometriosis and problems with her uterus, she endured month after month of excruciating physical pain. As the years passed and no children were born, her condition became increasingly worse and problematic. Eventually it became so severe that she was unable to continue working at her job. Her doctors pleaded with her to have surgery, the only option that would give her any relief from her symptoms. But she refused, instead choosing to endure the agony in her body and her heart. She was determined to not have the surgery because it would remove any future possibility of her being able to conceive and bear children. All of her hopes and dreams, all the days of her pain were wrapped up in her desperate desire to become pregnant.

Sadly, she never did conceive. Left devastated, she lost the hope she'd had for her happiness in life. Even in old age, she carried a deep sense of regret at never being able to create a child. You see, if like this lady your hope is centered strongly in the wrong place, it will eventually fail you, leaving you emptier and more dissatisfied than before.

Our dreams are like fine bone china. They are delicate and can be smashed to pieces with even the gentlest of knocks. So real is the fragility of our humanity that there is nothing in our lives that cannot be forever changed in an instant. Nothing is a sure thing, totally true, or able to remain unchanged—nothing, that is, except Christ and the inheritance He has kept for us. Only He can claim to be the same yesterday, today, and forever, fully dependable and alive for evermore.

Therefore, we must be careful of what our aspirations are and whom they concern. Right now, in this season of your life, they will most probably be linked to your strong desire to have a child and fulfil that natural ache in your body, mind, and soul. Even if this should come true for you, and your dream of becoming a parent is realized, it is still vital to learn this lesson now because its application is true for the whole of our lives. I have witnessed so many parents place a great deal of their hopes of accomplishment for their future in their physical children. If we are unable to see right now that our only sure and safe place is standing in Christ alone, no matter what our future holds, we will be in danger of transferring the fulfilment of our happiness onto something or someone else.

Take a moment to examine your own heart honestly and ask the Holy Spirit to reveal to you what or who it is you are relying on to get you through this season of your life. It may be that right now you are placing your trust in the latest reproductive technology, fertility treatment, or the promising statistics of your clinic. Your hope may even be in your fertility doctor or that little embryo sitting on ice, waiting for you. But what if those things vanished from your life tomorrow? Would you feel despair and be almost frantic about where to turn next? Or would you experience a deep-rooted stability in your spirit because your hope was never grounded in those things in the first place? No matter the outcome, the fact remains that relying on anything other than Christ is very deceptive, and what may seem like a pure intention could indeed draw our hearts away from Jesus.

When we give our trust and dreams to anything or anyone other than Christ, we will eventually become emotionally and physically exhausted. Instead of our hope sustaining us, we have to work hard at sustaining that sense of hope itself. Trying to prop up a groundless and idle entity is unsustainable; as much as you try to make it work for you, to make you happy and provide reason for your future, it can't. This is why you feel worn out, helpless, and disillusioned—because you are doing all the work for a false reality.

How wonderfully life-transforming it is to be confronted with a whole new kind of hope that has an entirely different way of operating. Instead of you trying to keep up your hopes, this living hope will conversely be the thing that lifts you up and sustains you. This hope is alive; it has a life of its own whose source comes from the very heart of Christ who pours it into you. It does not require you to give it life, purpose, or meaning, and rather than leaving you weak, it will pour strength into you in measures you never knew possible. Friends, in your darkest moments, in the saddest of days, when you feel like your hope is all but gone and you have barely enough strength to cry any more tears, I beg of you, collapse into the arms of Jesus and allow Him to comfort you. In these times, and I know it can be difficult; wait on the Lord, rest in Him, and He will renew (or exchange) your strength (Isa. 40:31). You know what is so wonderful about this? It's not that Christ will increase your own strength to sustain you but that He will give you a new strength from a different source. You will be emptied of your own strength, and He will transfer His strength into you. When you give up *your* hope, He will exchange it for a whole new hope that comes directly from Him. Your spirit will mount up with wings like eagles; you shall run and not be weary; you shall walk and not faint (Isaiah 40:31) because it is no longer you keeping your hopes up; it is the sustaining hope and power of Christ.

However, there is a catch! You can only experience this living hope if you have first been born again. "He has caused us to be *born again* to a living hope" (1 Peter 1:3b). Truly this is the most important question of the whole book that you must answer: "Have I been born again?" There is no point in trying to place your hope with Jesus for your dreams of having a baby if you have not first trusted Him with your eternal destiny. If you do not know Jesus personally, I pray that you not only question the source of your dreams but give them up completely in surrender to something, in fact someone, far greater, so much better—Jesus, our *Living Hope*. Without Jesus as your Saviour, you are not only living with merely a misplaced hope, but indeed "no hope." The Bible tells us that before we were Christians, we had no hope, and were without God in the world (Eph. 2:12). But when we are born again, we have a real, living, life-changing hope through Jesus. This hope can never die because as Jesus is alive forever, we can live in the assurance that our hope in Him will never die either.

For those of us who do belong to Jesus, I want to encourage and remind you that God has given you an unspeakably wonderful gift and resource in His provision of this Living Hope. I would beg of you to really take hold of it and practice more and more at placing every desire of your life into His hands and you will see how it changes the way you view your trials and problems. It will draw your heart more and more irresistibly toward Jesus and will refocus your outlook on the wider world and the people in it.

There is no doubt that, at times, it can be really tough to submit to Christ in this because it is just so much easier to trust in the physical. There will be moments when you will need to make a conscious decision to trust Him alone at the expense of everything else. You may find you do this for a time in your mind while you wait for your heart to catch up, but Jesus will honour this. As He transforms you heart, He will begin to show you little by little how futile it is to hope in anything else. There were times during that season when I found myself praying on a daily basis, "Jesus, let my hope be in You, let my hope be a living one because you are alive. Teach me, Lord, what that means and show me when I am tempted to start hoping in something or someone else."

Another passage in the Bible God used to really encourage me and help me understand this hope was the story of Rahab the prostitute (Josh. 2, 6). When her home city of Jericho was about to be completely wiped out by the invading Israelite army, this one girl, with her house on the city wall, trusted in the words of two Israelite spies for her life. She trusted that if she did what they said and hung a scarlet rope out of her window, then when the attack came, she and her family would be protected and kept safe in what seemed like the most desperate of circumstances. Rahab was placing her hope not only in her rope but in the word of these two spies she had previously helped. We've already noted that in our English language, we tend to think of hope in more abstract terms, but what's amazing about this story is that in the Hebrew, the word for cord or rope literally means hope! This story really helped me to understand that for the Christian, hope is very real and something we can actually grasp that is never out of reach. This was just a girl putting her trust in a couple of guys she didn't even know, but when you think about who and what we are putting our hope in, it completely blows your mind. We are trusting in the resurrected person of Jesus and the words of someone so much greater than mere men . . . God Himself. We place our trust not in the words of friends, family, doctors, or society in general, but in the words of God. One of my favorite verses is "I hope in your word" (Psalm 119:114b). That's why it is so important that we live our lives in His Word, reading it every day and saturating our souls with it because His Word is our hope, a sure thing.

As God's Word dwells in you and the power of Christ works and grows in you, you will no longer try to cling to a transitory hope; instead, you will be bursting with a joy that others will see and want too. This heavenly vibrant, sustaining hope will cause the world to look on and wonder why you are the way you are. They will not understand the deep peace and contentment you have. When they ask, tell them about it and about the person who not only gives it to you but can also give it to them (1 Peter 3:15). How amazing to think that even in this difficult season of our lives, we could turn this hope outwards to share with others as well as being deeply blessed in our own souls? I want to encourage you to pursue these heavenly treasures that will bring the deepest joy and satisfaction that words can hardly express.

An experiential knowledge of this hope in your present life will determine so much of how you deal with the highs, lows, and disappointments of your journey. You will wobble at times and be unsettled for sure, but your foundation will be secure. As long as you give up *your* hope in exchange for *His,* you will possess a deep-seated joy and rest that at times not even you will be able to understand. When the grace of God fills us, we are full of hope whether we ever get pregnant or not because the security of our future joy does not lie in us having a family but in the fact that Jesus is alive and we have an imperishable inheritance being kept in heaven for us. When you discover and *know* that He is truly enough, you will understand that in Him is the only true place we can find emotional stability, strength, and guaranteed peace.

CHAPTER 6

THE EMOTIONAL STONES

SOMETIMES, THERE ARE JUST NO words. Sometimes the pain is too deep to communicate. There are only tears. This is when I say, "I have 'the stones.'" It's a phrase Stephan and I use to describe that feeling that you get in the pit of your stomach when you feel like your world is falling apart, when it feels like you are weighed down with boulders and no words can articulate the feeling.

There are times when we need others' arms around us just to say, "I understand; I know; me too." I have felt these arms around me and have wrapped these arms around another. I have cried tears for myself and for others. As infertile couples, we shed the same tears for the same sorrow and own that we have no magic words or pat answers that will heal each other. Only we know the peculiar grief that is infertility and can read in each other's eyes the story of our sadness.

But there are stronger arms than ours that can cradle us every step of the way. There is wisdom beyond our understanding that will lift us above our own minds. There is a comfort that we cannot explain that will lighten the weight of our "stones" and cause peace to flood our souls. And all of this comes from the One who, because He shed tears for us, can now wipe away ours. Friends, this is our Jesus! This is our Jesus!

But let's face it; we don't always experience this or sense His presence close to us because our emotions can override so much of who we are. Even as we ourselves sometimes struggle to cope, it can also be very difficult for others to understand the emotional waves that crash over us. My prayer is that this chapter will help both you and those who seek to encourage you to understand a little more of why we feel the way we do and that together, we will all be strengthened in the Lord.

Over the years, I have read numerous Christian-based articles that could have been titled "How a Christian should *think* about fertility and reproduction" but not so many about "How we should *feel* about infertility." While it is vital we engage our minds when considering the questions surrounding this subject, the decisions we make and how we cope are fundamentally influenced and inextricably linked to our emotions. Like it or not, feelings play a huge role in the Christian's life when it comes to how we view our infertility.

The emotional state and emphasis of each couple will vary and fluctuate throughout their journey depending on their individual circumstances, personality, and physical health, among many other reasons. Rather than attempt to tackle all the twists and turns of the emotional roller coaster we have ridden, let's discuss a few very general aspects that affect most women at some point along the way. Please don't think I am excluding the men here, as if they are unaffected. Not at all. Stephan will help me out with you guys in chapter 13, but for now I want to focus mainly on the gals.

It is important to acknowledge that the strength of emotion involved in the pursuit of a child has the power to be nothing less than ferocious. When you hear a woman say she is "desperate for a child," she really does mean that she is in a state of desperation. Within the context of reproduction, our emotions can be so forceful that they drive us to think, say, and do things that at times can seem uncontrollable. One of the reasons I believe this is true for most, if not all, women is simply because barrenness strikes right at the very heart of one of our primal instincts for life and survival. When any of our basic needs (i.e. food, water, shelter, oxygen, sleep/rest) is compromised, then life becomes difficult to sustain at an optimum level. When all these basic requirements are provided to any species of living organisms within a controlled environment, then after a given period of time, they will naturally begin to reproduce. That is because physical reproduction, regardless of genus, is an automatic response within nature for the continued existence of any creature. However, when this deeply ingrained drive to reproduce cannot be fulfilled in the natural course of life, devastating consequences ensue. There is a sense of death and finality to the survival of that living community even when all other requirements for life are present.

When we then add to that the particular human dimension of emotional intelligence, any dysfunction in our reproductive ability can induce an even deeper level of distress. Our emotional and physical beings are so intertwined that they will often evoke a response in each other so that it is very difficult to feel dysfunction in one dimension and not another. In the same way that being deprived of bodily nourishment can cause distress to both the body and mind, so the physical inability to reproduce can have a deleterious effect on the health of our mental state. In 1 Samuel 1, Hannah "deeply distressed" (v10) by her physical inability to conceive, outwardly demonstrated her "great anxiety and vexation" (v16) through tears, while describing herself as "a woman troubled in spirit" (v15). You see her physical, emotional and spiritual being was simultaneously affected by her infertility.

When we are weak and vulnerable, it doesn't take much for these strong emotions to override our thinking and pull us down the wrong path. Where do we go when we are so broken and our only friend is grief? Will we ever be able to see clearly again through the heartache of yet another miscarriage? I do not in any way claim to have all the answers to a shortcut to resolve your pain or mine. But, God is aware of the depth of our feelings, and the Bible itself gives us a peek into the emotional turbulence experienced by some women going through infertility. I'm not going to go through them all, but there is one woman in particular whose struggle with infertility we can all relate to at least in part. Her name is Rachel, and we find her story in Genesis 29 and 30.

Rachel's emotional struggles were at times not so very different from our own, and there are a few key lessons we can learn from her life that may help us cope. At this point, it would be worthwhile to pause here and read her story in your own Bible. As you do so, ask the Holy Spirit to help you step into her world and reveal to you any truths He would have you see.

Rachel's life is an example of just how muddled our emotions can become regarding our childlessness and how powerful they can be in dictating our actions. Experiencing great highs and plummeting lows, Rachel appears to make many of her decisions based on her feelings, and she is frequently left feeling confused, frustrated, impatient, and bitter.

Right from the outset of her marriage, there's trouble brewing in this messed-up family. Seven years earlier, Jacob had been tricked into marrying her older sister Leah, believing he was marrying Rachel, the woman he really loved. Now 7 years later, after he finally gets to marry the girl of his dreams, a hint of unrest begins to surface in this love triangle. As infertility raises its ugly head, a perfect storm of hurt, jealousy, and distrust develops and continues to swirl throughout the rest of the story. Destructive feelings dominate their lives in the areas of sex and children. Time and again, the behaviour and words of these three characters flow directly from their screwed-up emotional states, resulting in a continual cycle of anger, resentment, and discontentment.

After years of being unable to have children and having watched her sister give birth, such was the depth of her sorrow that Rachel "envied her sister" and said to Jacob, "Give me children or I die"(Genesis 30:1b).

These words may first appear a little melodramatic, but when experiencing infertility, it is very common to go through a grieving process similar to that of losing someone close to you.

I remember listening to one particular girl talking about her experience. She said, "Every month when I find out I'm not pregnant . . . every time, I go through at least a two-day grieving process of where I literally feel like I've lost a child. Even though I know I'm not pregnant, all those days leading up to the day I take the test, I feel like maybe there is life in me, just maybe . . . you don't know. You start to believe there is the magic of a child growing inside you and you pray it is. And

THE EMOTIONAL STONES   103

then you find out you're not . . . again. The emotions I go through then are just crazy up and down."

This type of grief is very real and, girls, you do not need permission to feel it. Many, many women just collapse, head in hands, on the bathroom floor, sobbing from a broken heart every 28 days. It's not difficult for us to connect with Rachel's pain. It's not a great stretch of the imagination to believe that as she spoke those words, she literally felt as if she was grieving her emptiness and dying inside.

Not knowing what to do for her, Jacob gets ticked off at her attitude. Instead of responding in a caring and understanding way, he loses his temper and reacts in anger. "What do you think I can do about it? It's not up to me! Do you think I'm God or something? If God is not allowing this, then who am I to make it happen?"

[Note to husbands: this is *not* a good response! Jacob could have learned from his father Isaac and how he treated his wife Rebekah when she was having trouble getting pregnant. "Isaac prayed to the Lord for his wife, because she was barren" (Gen. 25:21a).]

I do actually feel a little bit sorry for our gal Rachel here because that's a lot to deal with when you're going through infertility. Perhaps a combination of longing to be a mother and envying her sister, with the added frustration of a husband who's not very understanding, is what drives her to her next course of action.

Seeing no way out of her situation, Rachel decided to carry out a little "reproductive intervention" of her own. As was the custom among some cultures in that day, Rachel persuaded Jacob to sleep with her servant girl, presuming she would take on the role of mother to any resulting children (v3). So strong was her desire to be a mom that she was willing to achieve it through whatever means available to her. Her identity was so wrapped up in being known as a mother that she behaved in a peremptory way rather than being thoughtful and wise. How often do we react impulsively when, because of our longing for a family, we rush decisions that should many times be afforded much more consideration? Our desire for a baby can cloud any rationality that we may need to apply to our situation, even if this means going against our feelings. This is especially true when approaching the subject of reproductive technologies, which is covered in detail in chapter 2. While we may smirk a little at Rachel's reproductive intervention "technique," we may find when we examine the motivations of our hearts that they indeed turn out to be just like hers.

Do we deem in our hearts that the outcome (i.e., having a baby) is more important than the means by which we achieve that result? We must be very honest with ourselves about these matters. If our heart's desire drives us and is wrongly motivated and not informed by our thinking and the Scriptures, we are at risk of ending up as Rachel did, emotionally wounded. ART is not something that you dabble in, but it consumes the whole of your life, and often the deepest scars left at the end are the emotional ones.

After her maidservant's child was born, Rachel was left feeling confused. I suspect she became aware that the fulfilment and happiness she thought her plan would bring her had not been realized. She did not experience the satisfaction she had anticipated, though she now had the baby she thought she wanted. Instead, she spiralled further into a pool of bitterness, strife, competition, and sibling rivalry that would affect the next decision she made in her pursuit of children.

Failing to learn from her first mistake, Rachel's drive to compete with her sister as far as having children was concerned was all the motivation she needed to persuade Jacob to have a second child with her maid. Messed up or what! At this point in her life, Rachel's actions were predominantly motivated by jealousy of her sister over even her desire for the child itself.

Ladies, this may seem a little extreme, but one of the most common responses from childless women is that of how jealous they are of other women who are able to bear children. This is true of many of us. Just because we are Christians doesn't mean we are not in danger of being consumed by this soul-destroying emotion of jealousy. I'm sure we don't need to search our own hearts too deeply for evidence of that burning envy existing within us. "Wrath is cruel and anger overwhelming, but who can stand before jealousy?" (Prov. 27:4); "A tranquil heart gives life to the flesh but envy makes the bones rot" (Prov. 14:30).

Our fertility is that one area of our lives that we cannot control; that area that just seems so unfair. Do you feel a pang of envy when you look around at the mothers in your church or place of work? Is it the feeling that somehow you've been treated unjustly when you see the young teenage mom dragging her kids along the street as if they were the worst inconvenience of her life? Then you hear of yet another devastated life of an abused and fatherless child, and nothing makes sense. Perhaps there's a little flare of anger that rises when the TV commercial comes on for baby formula or the latest family car, "perfect for all your little ones." Maybe you feel a little resentment every time you drive to the supermarket and the only space left is a parent-with-child parking space, and you think, *not for me.* You see, we are not as immune to jealousy as we might like to think we are. This issue is a serious one, and we need to be honest about how we respond to these feelings and how, if at all, we manage them.

When mixed with envy of other women, an obsessive desire to have children cannot fail to have a devastating effect on our lives and can only be handled and controlled by a higher power. In Rachel's case, the strength of her emotions drove her to seek out other ways of gratifying her need to become a mother. She thought it would not only satisfy the longings of her womb but also quench her envy and elevate her above her sister. So absorbed had she become with these feelings that when the child was born, her first response was to gloat, saying, "With mighty wrestlings I have wrestled with my sister and prevailed" (Gen. 30:8). How sad, that this is where it has brought her.

Meanwhile, Leah, now experiencing secondary infertility, appears to be playing Rachel at her own game and has also turned to giving Jacob to her maidservant. I think it's important to note here that even someone who has previously given birth often experiences the same heartache with secondary infertility as those going through it for the first time. The sibling rivalry in this dysfunctional family now seems to heat up as these two sisters become even more manipulative in their quest for children.

One particular day, Leah's eldest son Reuben arrives home from the fields with a gift of mandrakes for his mother. In ancient times, mandrake plants were believed to have magical reproductive properties specifically related to fertility. Women would sleep with them under their pillows in the hope of conceiving. So desperate was Rachel for any chance to get pregnant that when she saw the mandrakes, the strength of her desire once again became the determining factor in her subsequent actions. I'm sure she had no guaranteed scientific proof that these mandrakes worked, but she wasn't thinking with a rational mind. Despite having her adopted kids, there still remained a yearning and ache in her to be able to carry her own. All she was clinging to was the hope that these plants might be the key to her dreams. In her mind she had nothing left to lose, and so she struck a bargain with her sister and relinquished the sexual hold she appeared to have over her husband, agreeing to give him to Leah for the night. This was a high risk strategy for Rachel, because in doing this, she was allowing for an opportunity for Leah to conceive. And on that night, that it exactly what happened.

Poor Rachel, she just doesn't get it. On the one hand, she is entreating the Lord for a child. On the other, she is employing the superstitious devices of the heathens to help her get pregnant. She feels so powerless and is so mixed up in her emotional state that she is no longer able to distinguish between the power of prayer and superstitious nonsense.

While well meaning friends may not give us mandrakes to put under our pillows, does it ever frustrate the life out of you at some of the crazy advice they offer? We've all heard comments such as, "you just need to relax, stop stressing about it, and you'll get pregnant," or "you need to try taking these new vitamins." Then there's "have you tried standing on your head?" or "your problem is you think about it too much; just let it happen," as well as "maybe you just need to pray more." It's infuriating, isn't it? I mean, do people think we don't know every blooming position, cycle day, vitamin complex, and haven't prayed about it? Sometimes when I heard those I wanted to fire right back, "Don't tell me to relax! This is not a condition that a day at the spa is going to fix, and for all your 'advice,' I bet I could teach you a thing or two about how all this works! Are you having a laugh?" I'm sure many times my face has betrayed my thoughts but, girls, in these moments when our frustrations rise up inside us, ask God that we not be ruled by them and that we will respond with grace and then just take all that stuff to Him. At the same time, just because we know the difference between old wives' tales and the reality of our biological systems doesn't mean that in our desperation we cannot be tempted by ungodly practices and become confused about what is or is not okay to try in our quest.

Eventually, after about 7 years, we find that "God remembered Rachel" (Gen. 30:22a). At last, her yearnings and validation as a woman had been fulfilled and all her shame taken away when she said, "God has taken away my reproach" (Gen. 30:23b). Or had it? Now that she had a child, was she indeed fulfilled? I think not. Right after naming her new son *Joseph*, she went straight on to declare, "May the Lord add to me another son!" (Gen. 30:24b). I believe this statement was again uttered from a heart ruled by emotion. She was probably so overwhelmed with joy at the birth of her son that she wanted that feeling again. She wanted to repeat the experience because of how it made her feel and how it cemented her identity as a mother.

I'm not convinced that our gal Rachel ever found any peace and contentment in the area of having children and, sadly, when giving life to that second son she craved, she lost her own. It's kind of a sad story really, but it is a warning to us of just how twisted our thinking can become when our lives are ruled by our emotions when dealing with our infertility. As you read through her story again, you will be struck by just how many words relating to our emotions are in these verses. I have struggled with many of the same feelings as Rachel and at times have felt like that raging fire in Proverbs 30:16 that constantly demands more fuel, never reaching a point where it says "enough." Like Rachel, we may feel desires that will never be satisfied and emotions that will never be tamed.

But is it true that "we just can't help the way we feel"? Will we forever be at the mercy of the burning fire that is our emotions?

I can only share with you the words of another childless woman, words that transformed my life when I heard them and have since helped me deal with my emotions in many different areas of my life. These are the words of a mighty woman of God who went through experiences in life that caused her to feel the depth of sorrow at a level I cannot even begin to imagine. She is the amazing holocaust survivor, Corrie ten Boom. She said:

"In a forest fire, there's always one place the fire cannot reach.

It is the place where the fire has already burned!"

You see, when God gives us a heart that is already on fire for Him, it cannot be touched by the fire of the enemy. If we let him, our enemy will use these emotions to keep us from seeking peace in the right place, and we will be consumed by our feelings. He will use these destructive emotions to grip our souls and render us incapable of joy and useless for God's kingdom. The best protection we have against these raging emotions of jealousy, anger, disappointment, dissatisfaction, grief, and fear is to have the fire of God already burning with a passion and love for Him. That is ground the enemy cannot take. But for this to happen, we must have submissive hearts to Christ. We need to surrender our futures, our desires, our infertility, and what we think is best for our life and ask Him to burn in our hearts and to control the source and the direction of the "fire."

Friends, every time you become overwhelmed by emotion and you feel your heartbreak is more than you can bear, bow your head and surrender it again to Christ. Give Him your heart to control, and trust

Him with your life. Place all of your future into His hands. There will be times you may feel like you're running to Him every hour with this struggle as the enemy persists in trying to claim that ground that he wants to scorch. Don't allow him to do that! Ask your Heavenly Father to set your heart alight with His peace, having resolved to trust Him no matter what. He is faithful and will do this in you, and the treasure of knowing His presence and the reality of His peace in your life will become the most precious thing you will ever, ever possess.

If God has control of our hearts and emotions, then He will have control of our behavior. When we surrender to Him, we will be less likely to act out of our feelings, like Rachel did. Our decisions will be considered, and we will have a confidence in our choices. As you ask your Heavenly Father to help you take the right path for your life, He will calm your emotions and give you "the peace of God, which passes all understanding, [which] will guard your hearts and your minds in Christ Jesus" (Phil. 4:7).

The most amazing thing that will happen is that instead of seeking after happiness and never really finding it, like poor Rachel, you will instead be seeking after a person, Jesus, who is the only source of true joy. I encourage you to find joy in your journey with the words of the old-time minister, Andrew Murray:

"Do not seek gladness, for in that case you will not find it, because you are seeking feeling. But seek Jesus, follow Jesus and believe in Jesus and then gladness will be added to you."

This is my greatest desire for you: seek Jesus first, give Him control of your emotions, and let His Holy Spirit burn inside your heart. He will turn your mourning to joy and satisfy the ache in you in ways that no one or nothing else ever could.

CHAPTER 7

PRAYER – THE CRY OF THE HEART

PRAYER IS WHERE OUR BATTLES are fought and won, often in secret.

Prayer is what happens in the private place, in the moments when no one sees or hears but Christ. These are the moments we connect with our Saviour and Father on a spiritual plain, where we experience His Holy Spirit speaking for us when we have no words. It is in prayer that our hearts and spirits are in communion with Christ in a way that transcends any earthly communication known to man.

Prayer is the silent tear, the silent groaning of our inner most being (1 Sam. 1:13) and the mental, spiritual, and physical expression of our dependence on Him. Prayer is, in Hannah's words, when we pour our souls out before the Lord (1 Samuel 1:15b). It is the thing that will keep you functioning in the darkest of moments and make you sing in the midst of the battle. In prayer we will find calm for our raging emotions, and in prayer we will find clarity of mind.

Prayer is where we will fight these spiritual battles when our enemy would try to steal our reason and distance our hearts from our Saviour. In prayer Jesus will draw us close. We will know His presence, and He will speak to us with tender, comforting words. Prayer is what will lead us into worship and will focus our minds on Him. Throughout your infertility journey, you will need to pray for protection over your heart, mind, body, and marriage. You will be asking God to pour His strength into you (Eph. 3:14–16; Phil. 4:13) and give you discernment in all the difficult decisions you will be asked to make. It is likely that if it is not already the case, prayer will become a huge part of your life.

I cannot begin to tell you the place and importance of communion with the Lord in my life now. However, I did not always seek God this way. It was partially through our infertility journey that He began to cultivate in me a dependence on prayer that would grow into one of the greatest treasures of my life and feel as vital as the air I breathe.

Let's look at some of the precious lessons Stephan and I learned about prayer in this season that hopefully will help you too.

THE FANTASY OF PRAYER

How long have you been praying? Indeed, have you even been praying at all? Perhaps you and your spouse have been praying like crazy, maybe even fasting, and yet it just seems like no one is listening. Not only is there no sign of things getting better, but they appear to be getting worse.

Many individuals find the longer their prayers remain unanswered, the more worn out, despairing, and hopeless they become. They start to ask themselves questions like "is it even worth it anymore? What's the point? There's been no answer for so long. How long do I need to keep praying? Do I even believe God actually hears me? Is he not listening? Why doesn't he say yes?"

I too asked similar questions. When I examined many of the Scripture references to the "hearing and answering" of prayers relating to infertility, time and time again I read words along the lines of "and the Lord remembered [her] and [she] conceived," or "The Lord granted this prayer and his wife conceived." I couldn't find anywhere these prayers hadn't been answered with "yes" and a baby born.

How frustrating this was!

"Here we go again, Lord," I thought. *"Instead of your Word helping and instructing us, it's just doing my head in. How come you said yes to every single prayer in the Bible, and yet it seems like you're saying no to us?"*

As I began to look a little more closely at some of the couples that God had said yes to, the Lord began to teach me two very important lessons.

The first of these was that my perspective and focus needed to change in relation to my prayers. I realized that I was going to God as if He were

Santa Claus, asking him to fulfil my Christmas wish. He taught me that my prayers needed to change from constantly asking for a baby to first seeking after Him. He had to give me a heart that would "seek first the kingdom of God" and transform my mind to begin to want what He wanted for me.

During this time, God really had me face up to the deep idols of my heart and showed me that I was actually asking Him to fulfil my idolatry. I was definitely not God-focused in my prayers and was using Jesus to get what I wanted. Sometimes we just *want what we want*, regardless of what God wants for us.

Am I saying that we shouldn't take our petitions to God and ask him to "open our wombs"? Of course not. He wants us to ask him for these things, but first our request must come from a heart that allows Him control of the decision and that is prepared to accept the answer. And this is sometimes the core of the problem.

Are we afraid that if we invite Christ into our situation and allow Him to take over, He may want to do things differently than we would? What if He doesn't give us what we want after all? What if He wants to teach us that *He* is all we need? This can be a scary place of surrender. While we may think we want to agree, deep inside we are thinking, *I know you should be enough for me, Lord, and be my "everything," but if you don't mind and it's all the same to you, I'd still just rather have the baby, please.* As long as we keep Him at bay and don't fully surrender our lives, we will be living in "a fantasy of prayer" and will see Jesus as only being there to give us what we want, as if that is His purpose in our lives. The danger is that our love for Him will be dependent on what He gives us rather than who He is to us.

TO FIND HIS "BEST"

The second lesson I learned was that as long as I continued to think this way, I could also lay claim to promises that had never been given to me in the first place.

You see, children are given as a gift from God, but He never promised that we would all have them. It troubles my spirit sometimes when I read and hear comments such as the ones below.

"We have also been given the promise of a child. This is a promise that we are hanging on to. He knows the desires of our hearts."

"I thought because my husband had severe fertility issues that God was telling us He didn't want us to have children, but when I saw a sign from God, I knew IVF was in His plan. That made it even harder though, when my husband's sperm retrieval surgery was unsuccessful."

"We know it will happen for us one day because God wants to give us the desires of our hearts."

I'm not saying God cannot give you a promise or a sign, but it's not His usual way of doing things. God mainly speaks to us through His Word, and when we are basing our claim to such promises in the Scriptures, we must be very careful our hearts are not being deceived or misled. In the Bible, there is no general promise to us all that we should or would all bear children, and we must be careful that the strength of our desires does not lead us to misinterpret Scripture and go down a path that only leads to confusion.

For example, in Hebrews 11:11 we read that "by faith Sarah herself received power to conceive, even when she was past the age, since she considered Him faithful who had promised."

Girls, this does not mean, as I have previously heard, that as I pray for more faith, the more likely it is we will conceive. It is not a lack of faith that will leave you barren, and Sarah's faith was based on a previous promise that God had given specifically to *her*, not you or me.

God never promised us all the ability to have children, so don't put that on Him when He never guaranteed it in the first place. When God makes these promises in the Bible, as in the case of Sarah, they are usually very specific and given to specific people for particular purposes and times. Don't get wrongly hung up on thinking that if you are praying for greater faith, then God has promised this to you.

We can make the same error when considering the passage in Luke 11:5–13. We may think that the persistence of our prayers is what will get us the desired result. This error was illustrated in this comment made during a discussion among friends: "We must have prayed so much He finally gave in and said yes." But this is not the point of that story and is not always the way God answers prayer. Many have also used the story of Zechariah and Elizabeth (Luke 1) as an example of how continual, prolonged prayer is a means through which God finally "relents" or "gives in" and answers "yes." However, I do not believe this to be true in the case of this godly childless couple. By the time Zechariah hears from the angel to be told "his prayer has been heard" (v13) they are both at least 60 years old. This is one reason I don't think he was praying for a son at this time of his life or indeed had been for a long time. We must not assume that just because we pray repeatedly for a long time, that God has to answer "yes."

We must pray without having the answer played out in our minds. We must learn at this point in our lives to ask, "Not what do I think is best for me, but what does God say is best for me?"

You might see having a baby as the best thing for you, but that may not in fact be God's best for you. This is a difficult concept to get one's head round and it's even harder for your heart to accept. But we need to take heed and take some time to ask if it's God's plan for us to have a family, and what would He have us be involved in or not in our pursuit of this goal.

The question then is "how do we find out what His best is for us, and how do we get direction for our choices?" Let me take you to Philippians 1:9–10 and show you how He used this passage to help us with this question.

> **9** And it is my prayer that your love may abound more and more, with knowledge and all discernment, **10** so that you may approve what is excellent and so be pure and blameless for the day of Christ" (Phil. 1:9–10).

The Apostle Paul used a prayer to teach the Christians how to discern what things were "best" for them. In order for you to make the right choices, he says you need to pray so that you will have discernment when you look at something and know "that's what God would be pleased with and would want for me, and I know that thing is true and will bring peace to my life."

In essence, he says, "I need you to pray because I want you to make your choice or decision not because it looks like the best option but because you have been able to approve that it is excellent for your life." We cannot decide on something just because others say it's good for us. When the world, culture, medics, or even other Christians give you the green light but the Holy Spirit is showing you amber or red, you need to pray to be able to tell the difference between the "better" option and the "best" option. You cannot manipulate the Word of God to suit your own circumstances just because it's what others think is best if it's not necessarily what God says is best for you.

Paul wanted us to be sincere (authentic) and blameless about these things. Being in prayer will help you discern what is causing you doubt or uncertainty—especially when it comes to ART. If you have any uneasy feelings, being in prayer will help you know what is the right thing to do and will often change your perspective.

But how can we really approve what is excellent or best for us? In verse 9, Paul prays that their love may abound more and more *so that* they will be able to approve. As your love for Jesus grows and you abound in love for Him with all your heart, then this is what will help you decide what is best. If Paul can encourage you to get to a place where you love Jesus more and with everything that you are and have, then you will be able to recognize those things that are excellent.

In other words, your love for Jesus will affect your decision making. If your love is not focused on Jesus, then it will settle on self and your choices will revolve round what *you* think is best for you, not what *His* best is for you.

When you ask God, "How do I make the right choice for these life-altering situations?" the answer is "fall in love with Him." You see, if we love Him more than anything else, then our decisions will reflect our desire to honour His Word above all.

This though, requires surrender. Perhaps this is the day to stop choosing what you want, and in His presence, in prayer, surrender all you are and all your dreams to Him and begin to fall in love with Jesus all over again. Make Him the first desire of your heart.

FROM PAIN TO PRAYER

Over and over again, I have experienced how God takes areas of my life that had the potential to be a source of sorrow and turns them into the most amazing opportunity to serve others while being simultaneously blessed. This is no different for my prayer life, when so often I find myself on my knees to fight others' battles for them just as I fight my own. Together, we get to fight for each other.

For example, not too long ago I received a text from a woman in church to ask if I would pray for a member of her family. Nothing particularly unusual about that, but I hadn't known this woman very long. We were more like acquaintances who had met at a women's Bible study group that same year. So I was a little surprised when one evening she messaged to say that circumstances had arisen within her family circle that she didn't want to share with the church prayer group at large. She was just asking a couple of girls, of which I was one, to pray for this situation. She told me a close relative was very ill, suffering from the worst type of postnatal depression. The whole family was extremely concerned for her well-being and that of her baby and husband, and so asked me to pray for them all.

As honoured as I was to be asked into her world in this way, I was aware that only a few years earlier, I might have thought this request a little insensitive, given the nature of the problem. This girl knew Stephan and I couldn't have any kids and therefore might be unable to empathize with this plight as much as someone who had experienced it. Indeed, only a few weeks earlier, the subject of postnatal depression had been discussed at the women's study and so I was aware that there were people in church who had experienced this particular struggle. Would it not have made more sense for my new friend to have asked one of *them* to pray, since they could enter into what it was like? After all, how the heck could I ever relate to a woman having difficulties bonding with her new baby? I wondered then why she had come to me.

Completely unaware, this girl encouraged my heart by requesting my prayers, because she had recognized that my identity was not primarily defined by my infertility or having no knowledge of childbirth. I don't think it even entered her head that it might be an awkward thing to ask of me. Instead, she believed that if she asked me to pray for someone, then she trusted I would. She saw past the childlessness in my life and to my love for people that drove me to bring them before the Lord. She understood that my relationship with Christ was my security. The thrill in my soul of having the privilege to pray for this new mother and then getting to witness the happy outcome was dearer to me than my new friend could ever know. I'm sure she wasn't even slightly aware that the Lord used her to turn what was previously painful into sweet prayer and the most amazing opportunity for me to serve her unbelieving family while encouraging my own soul.

I have often noticed that the more time we spend with the Lord in prayer, the more He tends to refocus our hearts so that we don't become absorbed with our own needs and requests but have a desire to pray for others also. That indeed will return a treasure to your own spirit. How amazingly gracious is our God!

Friends, as you go through this journey full of potential pitfalls, God will answer your prayer, but it might not be the answer you were expecting. It would be wonderful if He replied yes to your petitions for a child, but if we seek Him first, then even if He says no, He will give you a different kind of treasure. As you seek to be with Him in prayer, just to be with Him, He will commune with you and establish a relationship so precious and trusting that whatever His answer is, you will be glad that it has been His choice and not yours.

CHAPTER 8

THE FERTILITY FURNACE

I'M SURE THE OTHER CUSTOMERS in the supermarket cafe must have thought I was either ill or a bit bonkers. My nephews would definitely lean toward the latter choice, but sometimes when God's Word speaks so deeply into my soul, my reaction can be difficult to disguise. I had finished my errands early and had an hour to spare before the school run. I took the opportunity to grab a coffee and read my Bible. As I was reading a very well known passage in Daniel, the verses just seemed to jump right off the pages and grab hold of my heart in a fresh way. The Holy Spirit brought those verses alive for the place and time I was in at that moment in my life. With my head resting on the table, I was overcome with the power of God's Word as it washed over me. As you take time to read this familiar story you probably heard in Sunday school, ask the Holy Spirit to allow you to see it in a fresh light.

This is the remarkable story of Daniel's three friends who took a stand against the powerful king of Babylon. Just to give you a little background, these three guys had been captured along with Daniel years before. They were from Israel's elite classes and were taken to Babylon, where they would learn a new culture and serve in the Babylonian government. God had given them great wisdom and learning so that they now found themselves among the top advisors to the king while still remaining faithful to their true God of Israel. This was a tricky balance, I'm sure, but they seemed to manage, until one day a new line was drawn in the sand that would force these guys to pick a side. This was no frivolous choice, for if they defied the king, they would certainly be sentenced to death. As you read their story from chapter 3 in the book of Daniel, allow yourself to be amazed at their God and His hand on their lives and destiny.

8 At that time certain Chaldeans came forward and maliciously accused the Jews. **9** They declared to King Nebuchadnezzar, "O king, live forever! **10** You, O king, have made a decree, that every man who hears the sound of the horn, pipe, lyre, trigon, harp, bagpipe, and every kind of music, shall fall down and worship the golden image. **11** And whoever does not fall down and worship shall be cast into a burning fiery furnace. **12** There are certain Jews whom you have appointed over the affairs of the province of Babylon: Shadrach, Meshach, and Abednego. These men, O king, pay no attention to you; they do not serve your gods or worship the golden image that you have set up."

13 Then Nebuchadnezzar in furious rage commanded that Shadrach, Meshach, and Abednego be brought. So they brought these men before the king. **14** Nebuchadnezzar answered and said to them, "Is it true, O Shadrach, Meshach, and Abednego, that you do not serve my gods or worship the golden image that I have set up? **15** Now if you are ready when you hear the sound of the horn, pipe, lyre, trigon, harp, bagpipe, and every kind of music, to fall down and worship the image that I have made, well and good. But if you do not worship, you shall immediately be cast into a burning fiery furnace. And who is the god who will deliver you out of my hands?"

16 Shadrach, Meshach, and Abednego answered and said to the king, "O Nebuchadnezzar, we have no need to answer you in this matter. **17** If this be so, our God whom we serve is able to deliver us from the burning fiery furnace, and he will deliver us out of your hand, O king. **18** But if not, be it

known to you, O king, that we will not serve your gods or
worship the golden image that you have set up."

19 Then Nebuchadnezzar was filled with fury, and the expression of his face was changed against Shadrach, Meshach,
and Abednego. He ordered the furnace heated seven times
more than it was usually heated. **20** And he ordered some
of the mighty men of his army to bind Shadrach, Meshach,
and Abednego, and to cast them into the burning fiery furnace. **21** Then these men were bound in their cloaks, their
tunics, their hats, and their other garments and they were
thrown into the burning fiery furnace. **22** Because the king's
order was urgent and the furnace overheated, the flame of
the fire killed those men who took up Shadrach, Meshach,
and Abednego. **23** And these three men, Shadrach, Meshach,
and Abednego, fell bound into the burning fiery furnace.

24 Then King Nebuchadnezzar was astonished and rose up in
haste. He declared to his counselors, "Did we not cast three
men bound into the fire?" They answered and said to the
king, "True, O king." **25** He answered and said, "But I see
four men unbound, walking in the midst of the fire, and
they are not hurt; and the appearance of the fourth is like a
son of the gods."

26 Then Nebuchadnezzar came near to the door of the
burning fiery furnace; he declared, "Shadrach, Meshach,
and Abednego, servants of the Most High God, come out,
and come here!" Then Shadrach, Meshach, and Abednego
came out from the fire. **27** And the satraps, the prefects,
the governors, and the king's counselors gathered together
and saw that the fire had not had any power over the bodies of those men. The hair of their heads was not singed,
their cloaks were not harmed, and no smell of fire had come

upon them. **28** Nebuchadnezzar answered and said, "Blessed be the God of Shadrach, Meshach, and Abednego, who has sent his angel and delivered his servants, who trusted in him, and set aside the king's command, and yielded up their bodies rather than serve and worship any god except their own God. **29** Therefore I make a decree: Any people, nation, or language that speaks anything against the God of Shadrach, Meshach, and Abednego shall be torn limb from limb, and their houses laid in ruins, for there is no other god who is able to rescue in this way." **30** Then the king promoted Shadrach, Meshach, and Abednego in the province of Babylon.

It's a great story, isn't it! I realize that none of us has been asked to literally go through this type of trial, and as such, their story is unique to them and should be considered the exception rather than the rule. I don't presume to place us in the same category as these friends, but nonetheless God used the testimony of these three young men to help us as a couple when we felt at times like the heat was turned up in our lives.

In a sense, every Christian who refuses to "bow down" to the world's demands will go through fiery furnaces of one kind or another. Whatever the reason, and if we are genuine, the fire will refine us like gold. We must go through suffering to produce any kind of character in us and lay open our hearts to reveal who we really are and who/what are the deep idols of our hearts. That being said, I believe there are specific times and circumstances in life when the fiery trial seems like it is "seven times hotter" than usual (v19).

For us I'm specifically thinking of the "furnace" of infertility, when some days you feel as if the heat of the trial has become so intense it may be impossible to bear. This is the day that you find out your IVF didn't work . . . on the same afternoon you hear your friend is pregnant—again. It's the day you are overcome with grief at yet another miscarriage. It's the day you wake up to discover that your natural time for childbearing is over, and you are overwhelmed with a fresh sense of hopelessness. It was during such days, when the emotional pain was searing, that I found the response of Shadrach, Meshach, and Abednego such an unbelievable comfort and encouragement to my soul.

These guys were full of confidence that their God was well able and powerful enough to rescue them from being burned alive, if that is what He so chose (v17). Theirs was the God of the miraculous and the God who was in complete control of every situation, no matter how dire and out of control their circumstances seemed to be. This was the God who created the earth with just the word of His mouth, so to rescue them for this furnace was child's play to Him, if that is what He chose to do. You know what is so amazing, though, is that this all powerful God they knew is exactly the same God we know, with exactly the same power to intervene in our lives. This is indeed great news for couples struggling with infertility; our God is more than able to do the impossible and can save us from this furnace, blessing us with children. As much as it excites my heart to know that we have the same God as these three friends, I believe that for many of us on this infertility path, it's the next verse that is perhaps even more significant.

18 "**But if not,** be it known to you, O king, that **we will not** serve your gods or worship the golden image that you have set up."

Hmmm, maybe this is not what you wanted to hear. I know there was a time I didn't want to hear this either. These boys acknowledged that the sovereignty and omnipotence of God meant that He could just as easily ask *for* their lives as save them and, amazingly, to this they were prepared to submit.

I truly believe that in order to get through our infertility trials and find joy on the way, this is also the place we need to get to. We must ultimately surrender our mind, body, heart, and spirit and be able to hear and accept the "***but if not . . .*" However, this will only happen when—like Shadrach, Meshach, and Abednego—our foremost desire is to put God above everything else. Our desire and commitment to honour Him has to be above all else that our heart desires and come before our very lives and that of any potential baby. When we truly see where Jesus must be in the equation and that His name must be above all other names, then we will sincerely worship Him whether He gives us what we want or not.

This is a truth that the Holy Spirit helped me to learn back then and continually reminds me of and teaches me over and over again now. It was during one of my "seven times hotter" moments that Jesus helped me to see this truth and profoundly changed my heart as He encouraged me to surrender to Him.

A FURNACE DAY . . .

During our preliminary medical investigations, there was one particular examination that I remember being excruciatingly painful, both physically and emotionally. When the nurse came to call me in for the procedure, she looked around to see where my partner was. But I was on my own that day as Stephan had an important examination for his PhD. Feeling sorry for me, she took me by the hand, led me into the treatment room, and gently explained what was about to happen. Lying in this darkened x-ray room, in the most vulnerable of positions, I was surrounded by what seemed like a room full of medical staff. I just lay there, praying, "*Jesus, please help me get through this.*" The doctor was struggling to get the procedure right and the more he tried, the more pain I experienced. Completely alone and feeling totally humiliated, I just continued to pray. The doctor gave up for a moment and came up to talk to me.

"Jo, have you had this done before?"

"No," I replied.

"Well, I have never seen anyone as calm as you going through this, especially with all the complications we're having, and especially having no one with you."

I could have burst into tears. I felt anything but calm inside, but I knew I wasn't alone; Someone was there, holding me together. What made this particular appointment even more emotionally challenging than usual was that, only two floors down, a friend was in the maternity ward having just had her "*nth*" baby.

This is so unfair, Lord; how can this be right? This was one of the few times I was really annoyed with Stephan, thinking, *Why do I need to go through all this and you're not even here!* My head was reeling with these thoughts when the Holy Spirit very gently invaded my mind.

"*Jo, I know this is a really dark moment for you, but even now I want you to have the name of Jesus above every other name.*"

"What a weird thought—where did that come from?" I asked myself, thinking I might have gone over to the crazy side.

"*Jo, my name has to be above the name of 'baby,' above the name of your fertility doctor, above the name of the latest fertility technique. Jo, through all this, you must keep me first.*"

As I lay there, silent tears slid down my cheeks as I surrendered all my hopes and dreams of getting pregnant to Jesus and into His care.

Two more doctors later, they eventually corrected the equipment and finished the procedure, and I knew I had had an encounter with Jesus that would have a rippling effect on so much of my future. So many times since, we had to keep asking whether Jesus' name was above every other name.

I felt that day like Jesus was in the furnace with me, as He will be with you, changing your heart so that He will become your main desire. You will need His protection more than ever, and you will realize you can only make it through the fire of infertility with Him right next to you.

BUT do not be deceived. It's important to notice that not everyone in the story felt the benefit of God's protection. The soldiers who were close to the furnace perished because of the ferocity of the heat. Even though these guards were not physically bound, they did not survive the flames because they were in fact in bondage by following the wrong master. King Nebuchadnezzar had control of their minds, wills, and actions; in other words, he had their worship! I have known of too many individuals and marriages that just didn't make it when the fire of the trial became too hot to handle. While you may think you are not "bound" in any way, you may be more dangerously tied than you think. When we give our hearts to anyone or anything other than Jesus, these things or people will not be able to save us when the trial comes. I urge you, run to Jesus, and you will truly know His presence in the furnace and will not be burned up.

A couple of dear friends helped me to see that we can place our full assurance in the goodness of God, whatever the outcome of our trial. Ten years ago their little girl was born at 26 weeks and weighing just 1lb 4oz; she wasn't even the size of her daddy's hand. The doctors didn't hold out much hope, and the next few days and weeks were a living nightmare for my friends. Then the phone call came to tell the parents to come to the hospital immediately due to growing concerns for her survival. As this godly couple prayed, heartbroken for their little girl and with no clue what the outcome of the day would be, T put his arm round his darling wife and, looking into her eyes, said, "G, whatever happens, God will do the right thing. I don't know what that will be, but I trust that whatever happens, God will do the right thing." What faith! But T was only able to speak these words because he had proven God in his life for many years before baby Beth ever came along.

Likewise, Shadrach, Meshach, and Abednego had complete trust that God would "do the right thing" no matter the outcome because they too had established a strong, grounded faith in God long before the fiery furnace turned up.

My hope is that first and foremost you make sure you have a true relationship with Jesus and then trust Him with all your heart! He'll never take you into a furnace that He can't protect you in. Just as the three boys experienced God's protection from the flames, it's when you're in the furnace that Jesus shows up in a way He's never made Himself known to you before. It's in those times you develop a relationship with Him you never imagined was possible. He changes your heart and gives you treasures that you wouldn't swap for anything. I'd go through this "fertility furnace" a hundred times over rather than go through life and never having met Jesus in the flames.

As you learn to lean on Him, He will forge spiritual steel into the framework of your very being, and you will know a strength like you could never have imagined. Then you will know it is Christ *in* you. I would urge you pursue Him first, entrust all your dreams of having a family to His care, and you too will find He is worth it.

CHAPTER 9

EXCEPT THAT ONE THING

TWO OF THE QUESTIONS THAT childless couples are eventually forced to face are these: "What will my life look like if we remain childless?" and "What will be my purpose in the absence of children?" The Scriptures came to my aid when asking such questions for my own life. The Lord also used a couple of key characters to encourage my heart and work through these issues.

One of my all-time favorite characters from the Bible has no name. This is the story of a remarkable woman with a burning desire to serve God in the place and time in which she lived. As I got to know her better, I was just blown away with the wisdom and kindness of God to include her in the Scriptures for us to learn from. Let's take a peek into her life to see how God placed her right in the middle of His work so that she not only survived infertility but thrived in the midst of it!

She is the Shunammite woman of 2 Kings 4:8–37. I wish I knew her name, but since the Bible doesn't reveal it, I call her "Shumi" for short.

Shumi was one amazing woman: smart, wealthy, hospitable, and popular within her community; in fact, she seemed to have it all going for her. She had the security of a nice home and was married to a godly, caring, hard-working man of considerable standing and influence in his own right. All in all, life was good, except for one thing . . . she had no children.

Right away, I'm sure many women totally "get" this girl and can draw many similarities between her life and theirs. Compared to a lot of people, you too seem to have everything going for you—great hubby, lovely home, amazing friends—everything, except that one thing. It may even be that things are so good in your life that you feel a little guilty for desiring that little 'added extra' of a baby.

Our girl's story unfolds as one day the famous prophet Elisha happened to be in her town, perhaps preaching or just on normal business. Gifted in hospitality, she decided to invite him and his servant Gehazi for dinner. She was probably a good cook and I'm sorry to say this is a talent I do not share with her! Anyway, during the course of the meal, Shumi recognized this was no ordinary traveler at her table. There was definitely something different about this dude, and when she realized he truly was a holy man of God, her heart was stirred to serve him all the more. So she decided she would help him out by giving him a place to stay whenever he should visit her town of Shunem.

I understand her desire to show hospitality to God's servants. However, if this was me, I'd plan to heat up a lasagna and put fresh sheets in the guest room. Not our gal Shumi! She wants to add a whole new, fully furnished granny flat/in-law suite to her house for Elisha just so he can have a private and quiet place to rest! Now *that* takes hospitality to a whole new level! Excited, she goes to find her husband to tell him about her home improvement ideas and get his views on the project. Being an attentive and generous man, he agrees and gives her the go-ahead for their renovations. Very soon afterwards, complete with new furniture and lighting, the new room was perfect for the prophet's return visit.

You can imagine how delighted Elisha was with his new holiday home. This necessitated more than just the usual thank-you card; he would need to come up with something better since she had gone to a lot of trouble to make this amazing new pad for him.

"What can I do for you?" he asks her. "I know some very influential people; perhaps I could put in a good word for you, even with the king or commander of the army?"

"Oh no, not at all," she replied, perhaps a little amused at his offer. "I'm fine where I am and quite content to be among my own people. Believe me, I've no aspirations of grandeur."

Somewhat perplexed and having no idea about gifts for women, a puzzled Elisha asks Gehazi, "What then is to be done for her?"

His perceptive servant, observing how down-to-earth our girl is, deduces that material possessions or positions of influence hold no great appeal for her. She has need or want of nothing . . . except that one thing. Possessing an insight into her life that the prophet seemed to lack, Gehazi gently makes the suggestion, "Well, she has no son and her husband is old . . . "

"Aaaahhhh!" exclaims Elisha as the torch flickers on above his head. "Let's call her up here at once."

Before she can even make it through the doorway of his room, an excited Elisha tells her about the gift he finally has for her.

"About this season, about this time next year, you shall embrace a son!"

In that moment, after years of continued disappointment, our gal breaks down, unveiling for the first time the depth of her pain. Could she allow herself to believe Elisha's declaration could ever come true? There is often nothing more hurtful to a person living with infertility than the words of hope from well-meaning but completely ignorant friends. In fact, it hurt so much that Shumi pleaded with this man of God not to dare say such things if not true.

You may be reading this book as a friend of someone experiencing infertility and are asking questions like, "What do I say to my friend who is going through infertility? What can I say that won't be the wrong thing? Is there anything I can say that will help?" I am frequently asked these questions by those who want to be sensitive to their friends' situation and want to support them. My answer is to ask the Lord for wisdom about what to say to your friend but give yourself a pass on this one. To be honest, there is very little if anything you can say that will help your friend "feel better" about infertility. The fact that she's opening up to you in the first place is an honour in itself. Infertility is still one of the most painful things to talk about, and so if she is sharing any of her trial with you, she is entrusting her heart to you, so count it a great compliment. This is also often an indication that she just wants a listening ear. She knows better than anyone that you can never understand her distress in this season, so don't tell her you do. Just be the friend that says, "I cannot even comprehend what you are going through, but I will be your shoulder to cry on and a listening ear."

Anyway, I would have loved to have been friends with Shumi. She is a role model for those of us with no kids for so many different reasons. Probably the first thing that struck me was the fact that Shumi is just an ordinary, run-of-the-mill woman like you and me. She is going about living her normal life in an ordinary town, quite content to be living among and serving her own people. She had no great wish to be anything special, but one thing she did have was a desire to be a servant.

It was to Shumi's house that Elisha was invited to dinner in the first instance. If nothing else, that shows she wanted to be around God's people, to learn from them, and to serve them. This woman was prepared to use what God had given her to serve Him, not focus on what He hadn't given her. She wanted to serve others and wasn't thinking, "Since I have no children, surely I deserve other luxuries in place."

Personally, I did think like this for a while. I felt like I deserved to indulge myself a little, almost as a recompense for not having the joy of children. Not Shumi, though; she was willing to use her "treasures" to serve others, not pander to her own whims. She was determined to be involved in God's work in whatever way she could, using the possessions and abilities God had gifted her. You have to admire her enthusiasm in doing this, especially building Elisha a whole new guest room! This young woman had the initiative to bring this about when no one else did.

The second thing I notice about this woman is her humility and consideration toward her husband. I love the way she brought "Mr.

Shumi" into her plans, showing him respect and not presuming to go ahead and do with her home as she wished without consulting him. I think our gal was in the habit of doing this, seeing herself and her hubby as one unit and doing life together. Her husband seemed to be somewhat older than she was, and she possibly saw in him a wisdom that she valued and needed. Some commentators have suggested this guy was a bit of a wimp, if not completely passive, but I don't agree. I think he was able to see right into his wife's heart, and as he recognized her desire to serve God's servant, indulged her in this and perhaps even helped her to do so.

Seriously, how cool does this marriage sound? To have a humble, thoughtful wife and just as considerate a husband—that's a dream to many people! Maybe I'm guilty of reading too much into this relationship, but I don't detect any bitterness between these two. In fact, I only observe a strong, God-honouring marriage where the love is obvious. At this point in the story, there's no hint of anything missing—we haven't yet been told that this couple doesn't have any kids! An important observation: we do not need to have children in our lives in order for us to have a great marriage.

The strength of character and humble attitude of this wealthy woman becomes even more extraordinary when we understand more about her culture. In those days, there was a real sense of shame that came along with having no children, especially for the woman. The fault was often, if not always, placed at the woman's feet, and so they tended to feel the greater part of responsibility and shame of being barren.

Such feelings are not all that different for us. The sense of shame that comes with thinking there is something wrong with you at the most basic level can become unbearable. The silence that surrounds you as friends avoid talking about your barrenness—while it dominates your thoughts—can make you feel like you are swirling in your own sea of humiliation and silent disgrace. No one wants to "go there," and the elephant in the room just reinforces your sense of brokenness and human inadequacy. Often, as a woman, no matter what you might say to the outside world, you feel like there is something wrong with you if you can't get pregnant, because that is what you're supposed to do.

I'm sure to some degree Shumi was not immune to such feelings, and I suspect she must have been all too aware of the stigma of being "different" to her peers. This alone could have been enough to send her into depression, maybe cause her to withdraw from her husband and community and resign herself to a life of perceived unfulfillment and physical meaninglessness. Living in her culture, she could easily have thought, "Well, I've failed in my role as a woman . . . so what else is there for me?"

Instead, I get the impression that this was a woman full of energy who grabbed life with both hands, not necessarily *because* she was infertile but *in spite* of being so.

Moreover, in Shumi's day, the importance of having a family, especially sons, was almost a matter of life and death. It was expected that sons would care and provide for their mothers in their old age. Women did not have the same rights and privileges as men at that time. Often, regardless of the couple's wealth when married, the woman was completely reliant on her children to look after her in the event of her husband's death. There was no such thing as social security or widow's pension, and Shumi would have been keenly aware that not only did she have no sons, but her husband was quite old. Her position was perhaps a precarious one. Infertility at that time often meant no hope for not just your present happiness but also your future security. This childlessness didn't just affect their present circumstances but had a significant impact on how they viewed their future.

Now you see why I find her remarkable. If this had been me, I must confess, I would have been thinking way into the future and building up a nest egg, just in case. I would probably have been fretting and wondering what was going to happen to me in my old age or even if I would be a young widow. While such musings may have crossed Shumi's mind also, her actions revealed the true thoughts of her heart. She wasn't hoarding or saving all her money for her future security in case she needed it; she was willing to use it for the Lord's work in the present. She was investing in His kingdom and not her own. She didn't build a granny flat for herself but a prophet's flat for Elisha to stay in. How cool is that!

This is just another demonstration of this woman's humility, where she was so focused on the needs of others that she was happy to serve without looking for anything in return. She didn't want accolades. Though her deep desire was to have a child, she never even hinted at that when Elisha asked her what she wanted. I don't think it even occurred to her to ask for such a thing!

I don't know about you, but most days I can only aspire to be such a woman. I want to encourage you though, that as you pursue your dream of having a child, don't make this your first or indeed your only consideration. We must be careful that we are not so focused on building our own families exclusively, but like Shumi we are investing in the things of God's kingdom.

Surely this woman was in so many ways an example of the Proverbs 31 woman, while not yet being a mother. I truly believe that whether we have children or not, if I have as much of a servant's heart and love for God's people as she did, He will give me work to do for Him. Christ will truly teach me what it means for Him to be enough, and my heart and mind won't always be unsatisfied.

Anyway, the next year Elisha's words did come true. Shumi gave birth to a gorgeous baby boy. And then they all lived happily ever after . . . well, not quite.

As I read on, I was even more convinced this remarkable woman should be one of my greatest examples to model because of her character both before and after she became a mother.

Take a moment and re-read her story in 2 Kings 4:8–37.

Shumi was a good mother and in no time her son grew into a fine young boy. A few years later, while out in the fields one morning with his dad, her little boy suddenly became seriously ill, crying with a severe pain in his head. Extremely worried, his dad arranged at once for him to be carried home to his mother. By lunchtime, he had become so sick that Shumi, unable to do anything to help him, cradled her boy in her arms as his little life slipped away. Very calmly, this extraordinary woman carried the body of her treasured child up to Elisha's room, laid him on the bed, then left the house . . .

If you don't know how the story ends, then I've left you hanging, and I'm sure you really want to find out what Shumi did next. But I prefer to encourage you to read God's Word, so I'm leaving the last bit of the story for you to find out from the Bible.

The one thing that struck me about this gal as her story into motherhood unfolds is that her character never seemed to change pre- and post- children!

I know so many women, including myself, that have been guilty of thinking:

If only we had kids, I would be so much better at . . .

Having more patience

Being more disciplined in my life

Being a more diligent worker

Having more confidence

Improving social skills and opportunities

And so on. Just fill in the blank for your life.

Not Shumi! Read her story again and you will see her character is sound; she didn't need kids to make her who she was. Her identity did not come from either her infertility or her motherhood. She was a calm, spiritually discerning, gentle woman with a servant's heart and love for God's people both before and after her role as a mother.

While there is most definitely a sense in which children can be the means to help teach us patience and refine our character, they need not be the only way. I would urge you during this time of infertility to ask God to grow in you a spirit like Shumi's: to develop and bring out in you those characteristics that will stand you in good stead should you ever become a parent.

Don't think that you have to wait to have children to grow in godliness and be involved in God's work. Shumi had no idea she would ever have a baby, and yet over her young life she had grown into a godly woman. It appears she never used her infertility as an excuse for laziness, bitterness, or an unfruitful life.

You can tell by her words and actions that she had the same humble respect for her husband before and after her little boy was born. I think this part of her character had a profound effect on how her household was run. I can imagine peace in her home, and everyone would know that "the heart of her husband trusts in her, and he will have no lack of gain. She does him good, and not harm, all the days of her life" (Prov. 31:11–12).

Whenever I read these words from Proverbs, I always have to say, "Note to self, Jo!" That's because I think it is so important for couples going through infertility to cultivate strong, loving marriages. I have seen so many husbands and wives allow their sorrow of infertility to turn into bitterness toward each other so that they end up forfeiting one of the greatest blessings of their lives: a happy, fulfilling marriage. I would encourage you as a couple to get before Jesus and ask Him to make Himself your "glue." Stick together and get into the habit of continually seeing yourselves as one unit, a family of two; that's just as important to nurture as any family of two plus. It takes just as much work, dedication, care, and vigilance to cultivate a fruitful and purposeful family of two as it does when children are added to the mix.

I think Shumi knew this and as a result had a strong bond with her husband even when there was no prospect of children. She was able to make the clear distinction between the role her husband played in her life with any role children would have. It's really important to understand that your spouse will never (and should never) fulfil any role that children would bring into your life. In 1 Sam 1:8 Elkanah made this mistake when he responded to his wife's heartbreak over her infertility when he said, "Hannah . . . why is your heart sad? Am I not more to you than ten sons?" Be careful, do not see your husband or wife as the one who will fulfil your desire or need for a child. It can be so easy sometimes to expect our spouses to fulfil our every desire, but they can't, so let's not put that on them. If you can separate your relationship with your spouse from any potential relationship with a child, I can tell you, it will save you from festering disappointment and blame.

One last thing that I think is inspiring about Shumi is that she doesn't appear to abandon the previous work God had given her once she attained motherhood. She still had Elisha's room; she never turned it into a nursery. It was on Elisha's bed that she laid her son, which would indicate that the prophet still used that room. I love that. It gives me confidence that what we are doing with our lives as we go through infertility is still valuable. Her investments in God's work were not just a "this'll do until I have a family" activity. No, they had lasting effects years after she had her son.

Friends, whatever you do, don't sit in limbo just waiting till children come along. Get involved in actively serving Christ now and be assured it won't be wasted or considered second best. Indeed, you may be doing a work that, should children be granted to you, you can bring them into with you.

My amazing sister-in-law Heather also reminded me that Shumi's strength of character helped her again when later on the Lord told her to leave her home because of a famine and she obeyed and stepped into the unknown with her son. Upon returning, and having to negotiate to get her home back, her reputation went before her, and the king returned to her more than she left behind. Heather said she just loved that the Lord gave Shumi more abundantly than she could ever hope or imagine. First by giving her a child, then restoring him to full health, and then returning her home and providing an extra income from the produce of her land.

I don't know about you, but that makes me really excited and hopeful for the future to see what He has in store for us and what He will have us do! No more limbo; let's choose to be a Shumi and get to work. Spend some time in prayer with an open Bible in front of you. If you haven't already done so, ask the Holy Spirit to reveal to you the work he would have you do as a childless individual and couple. Girls, if you are struggling with your role and identity as a woman, ask Him to help you discover what it really means to find your identity in Him and to give you a purpose in life that will have far-reaching effects not just for this present world but for the one to come.

CHAPTER 10

DARE TO BE AN ESTHER

DRIVING HOME ONE NEW YEAR'S Eve after dropping off some friends, I was talking with the Lord in the car about some things I wanted to be doing with my life in that season. At that time I felt like I was "fighting the fog" of confusion about what I was to do with my time, energies, talents, hopes, and dreams. During the journey, the Holy Spirit brought to mind some things He had shown me earlier in the year. Girls, as I share some of these things with you, you may also make some sense of what it is to be a little bit of an "Esther."

Begin by reading the short book of Esther. It's such a great story about a young Jewish girl who ended up winning a beauty contest to become the queen of the Persian Empire. Faced with what looked like certain death, this young woman went on to save a whole nation from genocide! Quite a girl!

After reading her story, I'm sure you have gone back and forth about what you think of this woman. One minute she seems a bit of an air head and the next a brave queen with nerves of steel. There is surely no doubt that Esther was one of the most powerful, influential women in the Bible and played a central role in the plan to save a whole nation of God's people and destroy their sworn enemy. Whatever you think of her, there is no denying she had some remarkable qualities: she was brave, she was a politician, she was a diplomat, she was a queen and a representative of God's people. But one thing is missing; there is no mention of Esther being a mother.

Not only did she not appear to be a mother, she didn't really seem to be much of a wife in the sense of the Proverbs 31 woman. She didn't have a great marriage or husband! But could we even dare to be the things that she was?

Ladies, don't be fooled into thinking that the only role or most important role for us is to be a wife and mother! While definitely a noble calling, don't believe the lie that it is necessarily the most valued or indeed the right calling for all of us.

This is one area, girls, where I sympathize with you when your life does not seem to be what people would generally envision as God's ideal for you, i.e., motherhood. We are often confronted, particularly in our western church culture, with the idea and expectation that when we get married, we should just automatically have children. The normality of this notion of how we should function as a family has become so ingrained in our churches that much of our church activities are created and scheduled around "family life," and by that they mean parents with kids.

Although unintentional, this notion of the "ideal family" only serves to underpin those feelings that if you do not fit into that category, something is wrong with you. The fact that millions of us will never experience this ideal is a sure indication that something is broken. The brokenness exists and God's ideal becomes redundant because of the result of the fall, the effects of sin, and the fact that we are affected by being born into a cursed world. You see, once we understand that, we realize that no human being is living out a life of God's ideal for them because, though the symptoms may be different, we are all broken and suffer different consequences.

In the absence of this ideal of being a mother, I believe there is another call for some of us women to be an "Esther": to be a strong woman in an environment outside of the home. A woman who will take God into a different arena with great wisdom, femininity, grace, and strength.

Is it possible that we could be missing out on a different route God planned for our lives because we are so focused on being the Proverbs 31 wife and mother? I suggest that you take some time and prayerfully ask God if this is what He wants for your life right now or whether He has tasks for you that do not involve having children.

I especially want you women who are going through or thinking about reproductive interventions such as IVF to consider this point. By the time you get to the stage of IVF, it often means you are consumed by the prospect of having a baby almost at the expense of everything else. When considering therapies such as IVF, we must be careful this does not cloud our ability to discover if God has other roles for us, and if so, what they might be. We must not let our identity be so caught up in being a mother that we are blind to any other calling God may have on our life.

Imagine if Esther had not been interested or active in anything else in life other than being a mother. If this had been her primary and only concern, it is possible she might not have been in a position to be used of God in the way that she was. This great opportunity to be involved in the lives of God's people and to grow immensely in her own faith may have passed her by if she had not been who and where she was at that time.

I'm not saying you shouldn't necessarily go through with therapeutic interventions (although this could be an option) or should give up your desire to have a family. Just don't waste the time you have now. Don't allow infertility to rob you of what great opportunities you may have to be involved in the lives of God's people now and to grow in your own knowledge of Him. It's a radical thought, but what might happen if you were to a stop pursuing one goal and actively go after other plans God may have for you?

Ask God to reveal to you where you should focus your efforts. What if you never become a parent? Does He want to develop your life in the world of work and business rather than in the home? While the home life is a good one, is it your foremost calling? Is that what He has planned for you, or does He want you to be involved in a ministry in a completely different area of life? Maybe He has made you the person you are, in this time and place, because He has other work for you to do, and with His guidance and help, you will be equipped with all the strength and skill this alternative life requires.

Being an Esther does not mean that we have to deny our femininity or charm as women; rather, we must be the woman God made us to be, even if that means going against the conventional train of thought. But then, Esther wasn't conventional at all! Maybe we have to risk our own dreams for His plans. Perhaps we are to be involved in more unstable or insecure situations in order to fulfil our calling.

I truly believe that God wants Esthers too; and so girls, if God asks us, will we dare to be an Esther?

CHAPTER 11

A FAMILY OF TWO

FIRST OF ALL, LET ME say I do not presume in any way to have all the answers for achieving the perfect marriage. I don't believe there is such a thing. I just want to briefly share with you a little of my own marriage and some of the difficulties we encountered and lessons we learned along the way. I understand everyone's marriage is unique; some of my friends have had very different experiences, but it is my hope that you will receive something here that will help you and that will make some sense for your relationship.

There is a plethora of helpful Christian books out there on marriage and family. However, many of these resources are written with the presupposition that, at some stage, children will be introduced into the family dynamic. The question then for childless couples with regards to marriage is "does this difference actually make a difference?"

My answer would be yes and no.

In many ways, childless couples have exactly the same relationship with each other as those with kids. Most of my friends and colleagues appear to experience the same joys and frustrations as we do. For many couples, whether they have kids or not, their marriages are wonderful while still being "broken." That is to say, because we have all been born into a fallen world, none of us will ever have the perfect marriage that God intended. In some respects, this means that striving to achieve this ideal state is almost pointless. Instead you are free to just be who God has made you to be, enjoying Him and each other.

Even after 20 years, the two of us love being together, and I reckon our relationship is not so very different from most marriages I know. No one gets your quirky little ways like your spouse does. I bet you don't laugh with others the same way you and your spouse do when you crack up at something only you two find funny. You're still learning new things about each other as you grow together, some of which are good and others, dare I say, not so much. Just the ease and security of being in your loved one's company makes life so much more relaxed and enjoyable. To be honest, you just can't imagine what life would be like without them and can't remember your world when they were not in it.

Don't get me wrong, though. While we rarely argue, as with every couple there are times of tension when we don't quite see eye to eye. Experience has taught us to keep short accounts with each other and never let discord fester and take root. It is true that most marriages will at some point be put under pressure and severely tested. The means by which this happens are innumerable and each couple's test peculiar to them. However, that being said, there are commonalities within particular trials that we can learn from and grow through.

The occurrence of infertility will force a couple to ask and answer deep, soul-searching questions that others have no reason to think about, never mind factor into their lives. There is no doubt that encountering infertility introduces a dimension of confusion to a couple's relationship and forces them to deal with unfulfilled expectations, whether they want to or not. If we remain childless, we will never be able to look at our spouse and share in that "she/he is the mother/father of my children" experience, regardless of the nature of the rest of our relationship. While many marital problems are introduced from an external source, infertility stems from within the relationship itself. This can cause a couple to feel isolated and alone as they struggle with where to place the "blame." If the issue is caused by their own selves, then does it follow that for the nature of the problem to change, they need to change?

It is throughout this involuntary process of change that a couple will either grow closer together or risk being driven apart. I have witnessed how infertility, with the potential to stretch the emotional and physical limits of even the strongest of relationships, has the power to break marriages. It is therefore vital that we do all we can to guard our marriages throughout this season of life, not so that they will just survive but that they will blossom into a beautiful testimony of Jesus' grace in our lives. More and more, I am persuaded that as Christians in this place and time in history, our families and friends need our marriages to work, our church body needs our marriages to work, and perhaps most importantly, the lost in the community around us need our marriages to work. Therefore, it is my prayer that some of the things we did and still do will inspire you to make Jesus the glue and the goal of your marriage.

A FAMILY OF TWO

The first thing I want you to be persuaded of is when people ask, "do you guys have any family?" you can answer *yes*! You see, when you and your spouse got married, you began your own family. You both became one: one flesh, one family. In other words, children are not an essential requirement for making a family; they are introduced into one that already exists, a family of two, husband and wife.

When Stephan and I sat down to discuss what to include in this chapter, I wasn't surprised that we came up with different things. We are very different from each other in so many ways. I know they say opposites attract, but in our case it's true for numerous things. Stephan is very sensible and measured; on the other hand, I have a tendency to be impulsive and more adventurous. Stephan is very wise with finances, whereas I usually forget to open the e-mail for my pay check. Stephan likes plain food, while I like spicy; he remembers birthdays and important dates, and I forget to pick my nephews up from school! He's a stickler for time; I'm such a scatterbrain and always late.

Okay, so we're both crazy about motorbikes, but sometimes I wonder how we can love being with each other so much when we are so dissimilar. But we do love being together, and I can't help but smile as I write this and think of him. The point is that while God has bound us together as one, he also sees us as individuals and therefore often works with us through different means.

In our experience, we noticed that when Christ brought us to the same conclusion, it was often by different routes. The following are some things Christ showed us both separately and together. It's possible that he will do the same with you, so don't be tempted to get frustrated with your spouse because they don't seem to "get it" or see things exactly as you do. They probably do, although from a different perspective. Recognize this in each other and use it as a means to learn from and support one another rather than as a reason for frustration to grow. I certainly had to learn this lesson since exasperation became my default after many of our early conversations.

IT'S GOOD TO TALK

It almost seems too obvious to mention, but perhaps more significant than any other aspect of our relationship is our ability to communicate with each other. While some of you may think, "surely that goes without saying," you would be surprised by the number of couples who struggle to communicate sometimes at even the most surface levels, never mind being able to discuss the deep issues of life. This is not necessarily a critical observation because many of us have never had this modelled for us. It may be that you are unsure how to share the deep insecurities, questions, and pain of your heart with your spouse. Perhaps you are afraid if you reveal your anxieties and uncertainties, your spouse will not understand or you will be in danger of adding to their hurt. I am naturally the type of person who holds onto my thoughts and bottles up my emotions, while Stephan is very open about most things in life and, as men often do, sees situations as black-and-white. In view of this, one of the key things Stephan said to me then, and sometimes reminds me of even now, was, "Jo, whatever we do, we don't go silent on one another."

If you haven't already done so, resolve to do the same for you both and open lines of communication between the three of you that will develop a deep-seated trust and safety in your relationship. No, it's not a typo. I did say, "between the three of you." As you reveal your hearts to one another and talk through these difficult issues, you need to invite Christ into your conversations. This three-way communication will become the cornerstone of your expression. His presence creates an environment of safety and dependency where you both will become full of expectation on hearing from Him and trusting Him to guide your thoughts and words toward each other. He removes any fear of disclosing any doubt or pain you think is too much to reveal. As you talk to Him, you discover there is no burden, no pressure, no problem in life that is too big for Him to cope with or to give advice and guidance on. He draws alongside the two of you and completely lifts the burden of your partner's pain being placed on your shoulders as He says, "Casting all your anxieties on him, because he cares for you" (1 Peter 5:7).

So much of the time, we try to struggle through on our own, relying on our own strength of mind and will when all the time He just wants us to give all of our burden and pain to Him. When we place our hurt and cares onto Him, our weight is simultaneously lifted. When you experience this together as a couple, you'll desire to make Him the focus of your marriage more and more and rest on nothing else but Him to be your glue. Jesus will take your gaze off yourself and lift it above even your spouse to focus on Him. Sometimes, He will make your soul feel like it is going to burst with joy and thankfulness that as you both sit in His company, you'll be so distracted by Him that you'll forget all about your infertility. As much as that might sound ridiculous, trust me, that's what He does, and you'll experience a thrill in your soul as He helps you to see your problems through His eyes.

HAVE FUN

This is probably one of the most profound, life-altering pieces of advice I can give you: have a laugh. I'm only being a little facetious because, believe me, you will cry enough tears together, so make sure you also allow yourselves to laugh a little. A lot, actually. Allow yourself to make jokes about your situation even when things are tough. Let your home not just be one of mourning but of joy and laughter as well. Life with infertility doesn't have to be all doom and gloom, and you will find humour in the most absurd things sometimes. Often, it's good just to take the craziness of the moment and turn it into something funny that will lift both your spirits.

Stephan and I have a whole heap of little phrases and quips that are funny to us, but others would think, "How can you laugh about something so serious or painful?" As much as the heartache can at times feel palpable, let the lightness be there too. Have fun together; just enjoy hanging out and laughing together.

A PRAYER OF PROTECTION

The more time you spend together with Jesus, the more you will realize how much He is invested in your marriage, loves your marriage, and wants it to be a blessing to you and those around you. It's no problem then for us to boldly ask Him to protect this union and rest in the knowledge that He will.

There were times throughout various stages of our journey when we felt more vulnerable than others. During these times, our prayers often became more frequent and specific, but there were a few prayers we prayed consistently and continue to do so.

The first was to pray for one another. Okay, I know you're thinking, "Duh," but while this may be the habit of some of you, it wasn't for us. We started to use our names when praying for each other, which made us really consider the needs of the other—especially when those needs were different from our own. This brought about a level of tenderness and thoughtfulness between us that hadn't existed before. By putting the needs of each other first, it drew us closer together. It grew in us a trust that we could safely and honestly open our hearts and know that not only would we not be judged but we would in fact be helping to fight one another's battles on our knees.

The second was to ask Jesus to protect our hearts and minds in relation to each other. As my dear friend Tommy says, "to keep our hearts sweet for Him and for each other." We asked that God would give us understanding for each other and that our hearts would be guarded from apportioning blame.

The third and most important prayer was to honour God in all the decisions we would need to make along the way. We were very conscious—well, Stephan more than me—that our prayers needed to be God-focused. Stephan would often say to me, "Jo, we need to be careful that we're not asking God to have His way in our lives and then just go off and do our own thing regardless." And so we prayed that God would direct all our steps and give us a real sense of peace that all our choices would be honouring to Him.

Friends, when it comes to your marriage, I would encourage you to fight the battles in prayer, allowing Christ to take control of all the pressure infertility can bring into your relationship.

US AGAIN?

Late one afternoon as we were driving home from a day at the beach, I became cross with the boys about their attitude. We had come to the end of a whole week's holiday of fun and now had to get back to get ready for school in the morning. It was beautiful, sunny weather (a rarity in NI), and the kids quite naturally wanted to spend as much time at the beach as they could.

"Why couldn't we just have stayed a bit longer? Sure there were loads of people still there!" they moaned. "You're no fun at all. It's just not fair!" On and on they went, complaining and pouting for nearly the whole journey.

Finally, fed up listening to them and trying to justify my position, I snapped, "After everything you have been allowed to do this past week, you are huffing because I've asked you to do this one thing!" I was annoyed as I thought about all the fun activities they had enjoyed that week without my stopping them even once from doing what they wanted. But now, in this moment, it was as if they had forgotten all that and could only see that they were not getting their way this time. All I had asked was that we leave a little early to give us time to get prepared for the next day, and they were being unreasonable!

As I think back on this event, I'm reminded that we as adults can respond in just the same way to our Heavenly Father when it comes to being childless. Stephan and I, at various stages, asked God the inevitable questions of "Why us?" "Not us again, Lord, how come things always seem to happen to us?" "How can it be fair that they can have children and we can't?"

You know, I think it is normal and only natural that you will find yourself asking such questions, but I don't think we will fully be given the answers in this life (and I don't think we'll care in the next one). But the danger is that we can become so focused on this one thing that God has appeared to say no to that we are never able to appreciate or even see all the things He is constantly saying yes about. We can have tunnel vision about this one issue and become blind to all the other wonderful things in our lives. Instead of giving Him thanks and being appreciative for all the amazing blessings He has showered on us, we pout and complain and agonize over the one thing He has asked us to go without.

Confronted with this, Stephan and I had to readjust our thinking to prevent the enemy from keeping us so fixated on that one thing that God was withholding from us in order to distract us from all the things God has said yes to, including each other. Every day it is good to be a little lost in wonder at what He has given us in this physical world.

We may need to have our spiritual eyes refocused to see that God had blessed us with all spiritual blessings in the heavenly places (Eph.

1:3) and, most of all, that we are blessed because we are in Christ. As your relationship with Jesus grows and deepens, you will love Him not because of what He has given you, but because of who He is. Ask Him to build that response into the framework of your marriage, and where there was once pouting, peace will start to blossom.

RECREATION VS. REPRODUCTION . . .

The inevitable subject of sex will come up whenever considering matters of fertility and reproduction. This is perhaps more pertinent for couples trying to conceive. It doesn't take very long before they consider their sex life in terms of the role of sex for reproduction and that for pleasure. The fact that you are reading this book in the first place is probably because there is dysfunction in this area of your life that could be considered the root of your problem. It is so important that a couple is intentional about staying intimately connected with one another, as the impact of this on a marriage can be hugely significant. I have considered this area of our lives in more depth in the next chapter.

DIFFERENT PAGES

One of the most challenging areas couples will face is that of exploratory medical investigations and whether they should consider artificial interventions. Every couple will need to answer these questions based on their personal convictions; many of these considerations were addressed in chapter 2. Therefore, here I just want add a little detail about some of the conclusions we arrived at in relation to our treatment choices and how they affected our marriage.

Stephan always had the thought in the back of his mind that if our fertility problems did indeed turn out to be medically significant, then we could always just go for IVF, and we'd be sorted. Ironically, once we were faced with this option and he knew more about it, he was the one who became deeply troubled about the whole idea, and he was the one who agonized about it in prayer the most. Although he was in agreement when we undertook the treatment, he was never 100% convinced this is what we should be doing. After much prayer and talking at length with each other, Stephan believed in his heart that before God, if this first cycle of treatment didn't work, then we should not continue with any more treatment. This was not a decision he made lightly. He was concerned that I would be angry and feel he was depriving me of the very real chance of having a baby. However, convinced this is what the Lord was telling him, he had a sense of peace that he was making the right choice. At the time, I'll admit I wasn't exactly on the same page, and although I wasn't convinced that I would want to undertake further treatment, neither was I persuaded that I wouldn't. In view of my feelings, this was a tough decision for Stephan to make, and so it was up to him to pray even more that if he was right, God would show me the same thing.

Stephan had a strong impression that should we decide to pursue this method of achieving our dream of having a baby, we would be stepping outside the will of God for our lives. He was concerned that if God kept saying "no" and we kept asking for a "yes" when that wasn't His best for us, we would be in danger of having one desire fulfilled but at the expense of another God-appointed purpose for our lives. He didn't want to make the same mistake as Abraham and try to fulfil a dream through means not directed by God and end up with an even bigger mess and heartache than before.

I had to ask God to give me a heart of submission and that I would allow Stephan to lead me in this, while honestly acknowledging my reservations. Through the Scriptures, God eventually brought me to the same convictions as Stephan. By the time we went to see our doctor after our intervention cycle had failed, we both had the same heart and peace about walking away from further treatment.

I tell you this part of our journey not to comment on your view of medical therapies, but to highlight the importance of being together on these things and to base your convictions in prayer and the Scriptures. Wives, it is important to submit to your husband's leading for these life-transforming decisions, even if they are not initially what you want. Help him to be properly informed and pray that he will "have the mind of Christ" and wisdom from above. But ultimately, if the deepest desire of both your hearts is to genuinely honour Christ first, then if required, no matter how difficult, let him have the final say and God will honour you in this. This was pivotal in our marriage because it was an outworking of how we were dealing with areas of idolatry in our relationship.

DETHRONED

By deciding to put what he believed was God's desire for our lives over and above my wants, Stephan clearly demonstrated that one of his idols had been knocked off the throne where God alone has the right to sit. That idol was me and his desire as a husband to please me, make me happy, and fulfil all my dreams. I guess this is the same for most husbands, and it is a commendable and noble thing to want the best for your wife and do what you can to see her happy. At the same time, what wife doesn't want to be treated in this way or to feel valued by her husband above every other person in his life? I know I did and for many years, Stephan indulged me in this while he gained much pleasure from being able to meet my wants and needs. However, when Jesus really started to get involved in the mix of our marriage, He began to turn a few tables upside down to reveal flaws and misdirected affections. I'll be honest; this can feel a little uncomfortable when He begins to shake up your priorities within your "family of two" and to expose the surface and deep idols of your hearts.

Up until that point, Stephan's priority in life had been my happiness and to do what he could to make my life as easy as possible. I was most definitely an idol in his life, and my needs and wants, including a child, came above everyone else—including God. Little by little, we were to learn the reality in our everyday lives of what it meant to give up our hold on anything or anyone else other than Christ. Over and over again, we had to take each other off the "throne of our hearts" and put Christ in his proper position, making Him our priority. The Holy Spirit gently revealed to us the areas in our lives where we had misplaced our hope and things we had given precedence to when we shouldn't. He opened our eyes more and more to understand that Christ was the only person who would ever be worthy of our worship.

Friends, if the focus of your marriage has become, as ours did, to have a child and a growing family, then I would urge you to ask the Holy Spirit to double-check for you how far up the priority list these things are. It is good and right to want children added to your family, but when this becomes your every waking thought and deepest ache in your being, then this good desire can become a destructive one. These idols will pull your heart, mind, and spirit away from Christ. Seen through to fulfilment, whether in a child or not, their empty promises will leave you more broken and emptier than you were before. If these things consume you, then they have your worship, and that alone belongs to Christ. As painful as it might be, ask Him to realign these affections so that together as a couple you will have the same goal, worshipping together from the same longing in your hearts.

SO WHAT NOW?

Just because we do not experience the norm and go through life without producing children, this does not necessarily mean that our family of two need not be fruitful. One of the most freeing things for us in our marriage was getting to a place of saying to God, "If having children of our own isn't what you have planned for us, then show us what it is you would have for us." Entrusting your lives to God and knowing that He has plans and purposes for you both is an exciting prospect. To be involved in building His kingdom, in whatever sphere He has decided, is an honour and rewarding beyond what we could ever dream for ourselves.

If God chooses not to include children in your future, please, please do not be despondent, but instead let your heart be full of hope for the future. Be excited at how He will use you to bear fruit for

Him in many other ways that may only be evident in the kingdom as together you build a different kind of spiritual legacy.

A family with children is a wonderful blessing from the Lord, but so is a family of two. Be encouraged in your own marriage as the two of you look to a future hope and grow in love for Jesus and each other.

CHAPTER 12

SEX WITHOUT CHILDREN

THE EVENING I SAT DOWN to write this chapter, I hadn't typed more than a few words when an old friend rang, in the mood for a good talk. With resignation in my hand, I closed the lid of my laptop, thinking, *I might as well forget about this subject until tomorrow.* Well, not quite. When my friend asked what I was doing, I told her about this chapter. Then, for the next two hours, she proceeded to "educate" me about relationships and the significance of sex in the absence of children, even though she has children herself. The most incredulous thing was that at the end of the phone call, she concluded, "But, Jo, I don't think you should include that stuff in your book. It is just way too personal to talk about."

Her response left me dumbfounded and rethinking my plan to broach this subject. I believe, however, it is precisely reactions like that of my friend that leave so many couples trapped in silent, shame-filled bedrooms of heartache. When a couple struggling with infertility voices any concern about their sex life, it is not because they are bored and need to rekindle the flame. No, these questions arise from a place of deep pain and suffering. These are very serious issues for the infertile couple and should never be considered frivolous or insignificant. Therefore, after much prayer and consideration, I feel it is important to address at least some of the sensitive issues surrounding this area of our marriages with the purpose of perhaps giving you a place to start discussing these things more openly with each other.

I admit, the topic of problems in your sex life isn't likely to come up in polite conversation, unless with your close girlfriends. Of course, I understand you're talking about a very personal and intimate relationship between husband and wife, but at the same time (and maybe this is the scientist in me) sex "is what it is." It affects so much of humanity's lives. It may influence the things that we do, the places we go, the conversations we engage in, what we choose to watch and wear, who our friends are, and often what we think. If sex has a bearing on all those aspects of our lives, why do we not talk about it more openly when it has such power for "good or bad" in our relationships?

One of the reasons infertility remains a taboo subject within our churches is because our Christian communities are just not comfortable with talking about sex, even in a God-honouring way. We may be fine discussing sex in the context of how it affects our young people and all the pressures they face, but we are no longer the young people and so are somewhat removed from the situation. Similarly, we have little difficulty addressing sexual orientation, because again, for many, this does not affect our personal circumstances. However, when it comes to talking about sex within the context of a loving, covenant relationship of marriage, where God has designed it to be, then that brings "you" right into the same scenario and experience as me. That is when it becomes awkward to discuss. Seems crazy, right? Surely if we can relate to the same experience, then we should be able to help one another with these issues that are key building blocks in our marriages.

I cannot comment on the sexual issues of those who have never experienced infertility, but over the years it has become apparent to me that for those of us struggling or who have struggled to conceive, we all tend to go through the same cycle of sexual turmoil, albeit to varying degrees, impact, and duration. There is no shortage of data to suggest that infertility plays havoc within your sex life, but you do not need to present the findings of any study to a couple to convince them of this. They would all agree it's a given that infertility equals dysfunctional sex! Don't think you are the only woman or couple feeling this way, because you're not. The rest of this chapter is not based exclusively on my own thoughts or personal experience but is a blend of many others that I hope you will find relatable and helpful in this part of your journey.

FUN VS. FUNCTION

We all know that feeling of butterflies in your stomach, when your heart skips a beat as you are first attracted to your spouse and in the early stages of your relationship. The stars in your eyes twinkle when you see them, and your sexual passion and desire are wrapped up in each other. At this stage of your relationship, the sex is more about the pleasure—the fun—than anything else. Among other things, our biochemistry plays an important role in our sexual attraction, and a cocktail of chemicals in our brains encourage this response and make our partner irresistible to us. This aspect of our love is a good, proper, and wholesome thing between two people within marriage, and it's gifted to us to enjoy by God Himself. The essence of the Greek word *eros* that describes the physical, sensual love between husband and wife is alluded to many times in the Bible (Song 1:13, 4:5–6, 7:7–9, 8:10; 1 Cor. 7:25; Eph. 5:31; and Heb. 13:4). It's important to know and understand that this is a part of our marriage that has been designed by God for bonding and pleasure and is important to Him. This has particular significance for the struggling couple when the *function* of sex begins to creep up on the *fun*.

As you begin to think about starting a family, the *functionality* of sex as designed for the purpose of reproduction starts to become just as important and relevant as the *fun* aspect. While still enjoying one another, you both now become much more conscious of the additional role you want sex to fulfil other than for pleasure alone. When nothing happens and no pregnancy occurs, you find yourself at the beginning of that road of confusion and anxiety, which often ends up in despairing sadness and conflict in your sex life.

As the weeks and months pass with no sign of conception, you become fixated on the idea that there may be something wrong with your reproductive systems. It begins to dawn on your consciousness that this baby-making thing is not as easy as you thought it would be.

A whole new flux of emotions start to invade your senses. Where you once enjoyed sex, you now start to experience just a hint of disquiet and even anxiety at the thought. Every couple knows that their emotional life, regardless of their biochemistry, influences and shapes their sexual experiences for better or worse.

The butterflies of excitement that once fluttered in your stomach have now turned into a little knot of nerves. The exhilarating anticipation you once felt has turned into a sinking feeling in your stomach of "will it work this time?" The stronger the interplay between our emotions and sexuality, the greater the potential these things have to affect our marriage.

As searing disappointment and emerging grief take hold of your soul, gripping you tighter every 28 days, the dysfunction of sex overshadows everything else that God designed it to be. Both of you are now so focused on your emptiness that what was once a beautiful thing that brought you closer together has now just become a reminder of your "brokenness."

Sex for reproduction can overpower everything else at this stage. A couple in pursuit of a child will do everything they can to optimize the chances of getting pregnant. Gone are the days of spontaneity and romantic surprises, as their sex life is planned and timed with military precision around the wife's cycle. Sex needs to happen at specific times on specific days, and so it can become almost mechanical in the absence of passion. At this stage of the game, function overrides pleasure, and the mechanics become more important than any bonding that may happen between the two of you. From a medical perspective, this is the correct approach to take and is advocated when trying to get pregnant but with it comes a hidden biological source of distress. What was once a thing that brought you both happiness and satisfaction has now become the very thing that has introduced frustration, anxiety, and disappointment.

The lack of concordance that now exists between the two main roles of sex becomes ever more reinforced in our minds, bodies, and spirits as the months begin to turn into years. The feeling of hopelessness can become overwhelming as the cycle of built-up hope—that each time you have sex might just be the one that works—is crushed every month when you find out you're not pregnant. Anticipating sex, you find yourself asking, "What's the point? Not only is this not fun, it's not fit for any other reason."

I think we are given an illustration in Genesis 30:14–15 showing this change in how we view sex in terms of for pleasure or procreation is common, especially in women. At this stage of Rachel's infertility journey, her behavior would indicate that the purpose of sex for having children was more important to her than having her husband in her bed, full stop. Hers was a complicated marriage where the other wife, Leah, was also her sister. Rachel was the sister to whom Jacob was attracted, and so it would appear her bed is where he spent his nights. When one day Leah came into possession of mandrake plants that were thought to promote fertility, Rachel jumped at the chance to get hold of them, such was her desire to conceive. In exchange for the mandrakes, she gave Jacob to Leah for the night. Most likely she told herself, "I can have him anytime I want. No big deal in giving him to Leah for a night, because when he returns to my bed, I'll have the mandrakes and their power to help me conceive." It is obvious here that Rachel viewed sex more in terms of reproduction than recreation, which I would suggest would become even more reinforced the longer her infertility continued.

These are intimate reflections, I know, but any couple dealing with these issues will be able to relate to the reality of what it's like to live through. The strain that this puts on marriages is huge and can be used by the devil to drive a wedge between the couple (1 Cor. 7:5), making sex an emotionally painful experience rather than a good one. The collision of these two aspects of sex can become seriously problematic and have a damaging effect on not only a couple's physical relationship but the whole of their life together.

I think it is fair to say that if or when reproductive interventions such as IVF/ICSI are introduced, they bring with them an avalanche of hormonally induced emotions and physical ordeals so that any distress and complications experienced up until this point are increased exponentially. It is no exaggeration to say that there are times when you feel your sex life *is* your life, and not in a good way. In trying to fix the functionality of sex, our whole lives become consumed by it and the need for it "to work."

Now it becomes a little more understandable why many infertile Christian couples feel isolated and unable to find support within their church. While their thoughts are constantly occupied with sex, no one else wants to talk about it! These couples don't necessarily want to share the intimate details of their love life with everyone, but they would likely appreciate others understanding or being aware of the impact of such things that have a profound bearing on who they are as a person during that season of their life.

BONDING: BIBLICAL OR BIOLOGICAL?

Scientific evidence suggests that not only does our brain biochemistry play a role in our initial attraction to one another, i.e., through the release of "reward" chemicals such as the neurotransmitter dopamine, but also that hormones such as "the cuddle hormone" oxytocin play an important role in promoting bonding between individuals and cementing long-term relationships.

The transition and levels of such chemicals throughout the progression of a relationship change. Some have suggested that as the role of the reward's hormones diminishes, the impact of the bonding or "cuddle" hormones become more important. Often by the time a couple's "honeymoon period" is over, they have additional reasons to bond them together, as well as increased levels of bonding hormones—one reason being children. The birth of children is also thought to strengthen relationships in part by the release and increased levels of bonding hormones such as oxytocin. Even when it seems the passion has cooled between a couple, there is evidence to suggest that despite that, they remain attached because of their children. How many times have I heard comments such as "The only reason I don't leave this marriage is because I couldn't walk out on my kids," or "I'm just sticking it out with him/her for the sake of the kids."

While we cannot attribute all, or even the majority, of our feelings and decisions to our biochemistry, it is true that they do play a significant role. So what happens when the natural progression of both our sexual and bonding hormones is interrupted, as may be the case for infertile couples? What bonds us together in long-term relationships where there are no kids involved?

For some, the prospect of lack of fulfilment becomes too big a wedge that ends up driving the couple apart and ending the marriage. For others, the lack of stimulation and absence of anything else to keep them committed has driven them to find fulfilment, whether that be in terms of function or fun, in another's arms.

So if there are no children, are we more susceptible to stray or to go looking for another life? Are we more likely to be tempted by another because we perceive we have less to lose and therefore the risk not as great? Do we tend to drift into separate lives, especially in our careers and friendships? Just because we are Christians does not make us immune to these things. These are real issues that should be discussed openly and honestly, especially if you are at the stage in your journey where it is likely that having kids is no longer a probability.

These are serious issues that if left unresolved can have devastating effects within a marriage. I have witnessed the heartbreak of individuals and the devastation their infertility left behind, leaving carnage in its wake, breaking up marriages, and stealing the opportunity for a wonderful relationship even in the absence of children. I know of sexless marriages that have remained that way for years because the pain introduced through infertility has never been resolved. These things not only destroy lives but also break the very heart of God, and, friends, this is not what He wants for us. Therefore, it is important for the infertile couple to be vigilant about the area of their sex life and be careful to nurture what God would have intended for them.

While many couples are indeed able to resume some semblance of a nourishing, fulfilling intimate relationship, I suggest that for the rest of you struggling, there is a restorative path that God has provided for us.

God may never restore the reproductive function of sex for you—that's His choice—but He does desire that we nurture it in our marriages for all other reasons outside of making a baby. Our Heavenly Father knows how difficult an area this can be for us and, seeing our hurt, wants to redeem our sex lives and give us a close relationship with each other that will be a wonderful blessing to us and be honouring to Him.

We need to take this pain and dysfunction to Him and say, "Lord, this sucks, and I don't know how to fix it, but I know you do, and I give all this to you, trusting that you know what to do." God takes what is broken and puts it back together His way and gives you something even more special, tender, and beautiful than anything you had before. How He redeems and restores your intimate relationship with one another will be different, I'm sure, for each individual couple, but every time we surrender this part of our lives to Him, He will honour that and protect and bless you in it. There is no doubt this will be a difficult season in that respect, but it will not always be that way. If both of you depend on Jesus and stay close to Him as you walk this path, He will guard you both, and as together you endeavour to draw nearer to Him, you will simultaneously be drawn closer to each other.

CHAPTER 13

AN EMPTY QUIVER

ACCORDING TO THE BIBLE, A man's children are one of his life's greatest treasures and blessings. What a joy these children are to him as described in the words of Psalm 127:3–5:

3 Behold, children are a heritage from the Lord,

The fruit of the womb a reward.

4 Like arrows in the hand of a warrior

Are the children of one's youth.

5 Blessed is the man who fills his quiver with them!

He shall not be put to shame

When he speaks with his enemies in the gate.

How wonderful, what a sense of achievement and contented fulfilment these words convey. Very happy is this man who possesses a "quiver full of arrows." But not so for our men while their quiver remains empty and their part in this blessing denied.

Men don't often talk about infertility. Rarely do they find themselves discussing this topic with their friends or colleagues. Sometimes, our husbands even find it difficult to open up to us about how they are coping and truly feeling in respect to these issues. But, guys, we recognize that you are one half of our marriages and that childlessness affects you as much as it does us. As a woman, I cannot represent you fairly, and so for the most part this chapter is Stephan's words and thoughts. In sharing some of his personal reflections, we pray that you men would be encouraged and your spirit strengthened during this season of your life.

When I asked Stephan what the most difficult thing was about his journey, without hesitation he answered, "Having to watch you suffer."

As a husband the hardest thing for him was to watch the disappointment his wife went through, experiencing month after month of no pregnancy.

"I could only cradle you in my arms as you cried while I felt so helpless to do anything to take away your pain. It was all I could do to keep from weeping with you—or more for you—but I wouldn't allow my tears to come. I knew I needed to be strong for you and be there to console you. I needed to let you grieve but inside, I grieved with you."

He then went on to explain that he felt many times that he had to put his own feelings aside because, no matter how sad or guilty he felt, he wanted to absorb as much of my pain as he could instead of laying any more on me. Whatever was going on with him, he felt first and foremost that he needed to be my support and comfort.

Another area of our journey where Stephan felt he was able to shoulder some of the emotional turmoil was by considering himself the one with the physical problem. He reasoned that with all the bodily hurt I experienced, whether through fertility treatments or just the monthly cycle, the extra emotional burden I might place on myself would be too much for me to bear. Therefore, he was glad to be the one to bear any sense of guilt and shame that came along with that.

My heart breaks a little at this because, although I will never know, he may actually have been right in his assessment of my emotional and mental state of mind. I never considered how this issue might apply to me and also admit I never gave it enough consideration for Stephan either. We prayed loads about this particular area of our relationship, for our hearts and minds to be protected from portioning any blame for our inability to conceive, and for us to see our infertility as a joint issue, never the problem of a single person. Still, although we confronted these issues together, his perception of being at fault came with a real sense of guilt and shame. Indeed, some couples acknowledge that they wouldn't be able to cope with knowing who, if either, was to blame for their infertility and therefore refrain from undertaking any medical investigations.

The guilt he felt stemmed from his feelings of inadequacy due to being unable to make my dreams of having our own children come true. He also felt like we'd had to overcome so many hurdles at the beginning of our marriage due to his physical injuries, so our ongoing infertility issues compounded those feelings of guilt. Our physical inability to conceive without intervention left him feeling like he wasn't a "real man," able to fulfil even the basic functions of life.

From conversations he has had with a number of men in the same position, he relayed that this sense of shame of feeling as if you were not fulfilling your role as man exists with many men. Many men feel isolated within their circle of family and friends because all the sympathy seems to be directed toward the wife and what she must go through physically as well as emotionally. Frustration can arise because men remain silent, thinking to themselves, "Just because we don't show it or don't carry the baby doesn't mean we don't suffer the emotional effects too."

When I asked Stephan how he dealt with these issues and what helped him, he answered, "in much of it Jo, you helped me. You never made me feel like I had done you any wrong, and any guilt I felt wasn't because it came from you. When Jesus took your anxiety away, all the blame I felt was gone too."

Ladies, this is a huge compliment to be paid from our husbands. It's so important that we ask the Lord to help us help our men and to be wise in what we say and how we react. Our words betray our hearts, and so we need to be in communion with Christ for the words to say before we talk to our husbands. They are suffering also. We need to ask Jesus to use this to draw us closer together so that there is no opportunity for resentment to take root and bitterness to grow.

I went on to ask him, "So if you were to give some other young man any advice for how to get through this season of his life with joy and be a good husband to his wife, what would you say?"

"Pray. Pray with your wife and pray for your wife. Pray for your marriage and pray for yourself. Then pray again." He then reminded me of the example of Isaac's response to Rebekah when they couldn't get pregnant. "Isaac prayed to the Lord for his wife, because she was barren" (Gen. 25:21a). Similarly, in Luke 1, Zechariah response to his wife's barrenness was to rely on prayer.

I laughed when he said this, because whenever a problem arises, the first thing he usually says to me is, "Jo, shall we just pray?" I should've guessed this is what he'd say when I asked.

I had to coax him a little more for these further few points:

"Listen." Just being there to listen to your wife is one of the most important things you can do for her. No matter how silly or unreasonable things she says may sound, the fact is that's how she feels in that moment. Women often need to process their thoughts by talking through them, so serve her by being a listening ear whenever she needs it.

Talk to your wife and express your own fears as well as being prepared to accept hers.

Don't say, "It doesn't really matter," or "we can try again next month." This can be devastating to your wife and might convey that you don't really care even, when nothing could be further from the truth. Men tend to see things more in black-and-white, while women take longer to process their feelings. For example, Stephan said that he was able to move on much more quickly every month than I did. He said men need to recognize this and be very sensitive in what they say and how they say it.

Constantly reassure your wife and never ever give any sense of apportioning blame. Be strong for her. Every time you think your own pain is searing, imagine it is even worse for her and you'll have no problem putting her needs before your own.

Understand that the dynamics of your physical, intimate relationship will change for a time. You will need to be constantly trying to be aware of where your wife is emotionally and physically in this respect. Put your wife's needs first during this time and ask God to give you all the wisdom you will need.

Be careful never to speak rashly to your wife, especially in moments of frustration, vulnerability, or weakness. In Genesis 30:1–2 Jacob reacted this way to Rachel, which only inflicted more pain on her and contributed to her making wrong choices in the future. "There is one whose rash words are like sword thrusts, but the tongue of the wise brings healing" (Prov. 12:18).

Make sure that before you make any decision about your life as a couple, you realize you as the husband must take responsibility for you both. Make sure you pray and are guided by the Bible and that you have a real sense of peace from the Lord before you do anything.

Make your wife laugh. Nothing will lift your day more than seeing your wife smile.

To our men whose quivers yet remain empty, let us share with you one of our favorite men from the Bible who has been an inspiration to us, as he lived his life most probably experiencing involuntary infertility.

As a handsome, fit, and intelligent young man from a noble family, Daniel had been taken captive by King Nebuchadnezzar into Babylon. By selecting the best of the young men, the king's intent was to assimilate them into the way of life and customs of their new country so that their captors would ultimately benefit from their learning and skills. God chose to give Daniel a special ability to learn and skilled him in all literature and wisdom. Recognizing his qualities, the king eventually appointed him as one of his most senior and trusted advisors. Only one problem. This meant that Daniel would spend much of his time in and around the palace, where not only the king lived but also his wives and harem. Concerned with his heirs being genuine, the last thing the king wanted around "his women" were handsome young men. Therefore, in order to protect his line while still having access to his advisors, these young men were castrated.

Others have also suggested that Daniel and his friends may indeed already have been eunuchs before they were even captured. While the Scriptures don't give us explicit details that this is what happened to Daniel, it is implied.

We never read of Daniel having a wife or children. In addition, when threatened with death, no mention follows of this punishment befalling his family, as was the custom in those days. There is no mention in Scripture or history books of offspring Daniel may have had, and given his position it is highly likely that he lived as a eunuch for the majority of his life.

However, there is no doubt that God had very important and specific plans for Daniel's life outside of having his own natural family. God placed him in a high position of influence that would often be precarious and high risk, right at the center of the heathen Babylonian empire. And yet throughout his whole life, Daniel impresses us as a man with a servant's heart, honoured to even be involved in God's work, no matter what it looked like for his life. He was a man of prayer and humility, whose heart remained tender toward his God from his youngest days to his oldest. His life, will, and mind were taken up with serving and worshipping God and serving those around him.

Even as a young man, Daniel's mindset was one of surrender and submission to God. Never do we read of him huffing or pouting because of what God has asked him to forego by placing him in the position he had. I wonder sometimes what Daniel prayed about or prayed for when he opened his window three times every day (Daniel 6:10). Was he praying that God would change his circumstances in life? I have no idea, and though we know that he prayed specifically for things, he also "got down on his knees . . . and gave thanks before his God, as he had done previously" (Daniel 6:10b). I wonder what he was giving thanks for. It doesn't really matter. What's important is that over the course of his life and throughout all his trials, God has placed in him a thankful heart! There is no hint that he believed his position or work was second best or that he had missed out on anything. No, even in his senior years, his heart was to bless the Lord who had been so gracious to him.

Guys, even if your quiver remains empty, like Daniel, how amazing would it be to reach your twilight years and see that you have known and experienced God's grace in powerful ways as you walked with Him? To find your heart is only filled with thankfulness toward Him? No disappointment, no feeling of having been denied this blessing of children, but instead rejoicing for having been given everything you didn't deserve, His grace in your life.

No one can deny the impact Daniel's life had on history and on the people around Him. Daniel may not have left a physical lineage, but my, did he ever leave a legacy. Not only did Daniel have a powerful impact on the Babylonians but also on his own countrymen and his friends Shadrach, Meshach, and Abednego. This little band of childless men turned their world upside down and steered the course of history for the very country that held them captive.

Friends, the next time your heart is feeling deprived and the words, "why me?" form on your lips, stop and consider that maybe the Lord has another work for you to do. We don't always like how our lives are playing out, but it is His script to write. While we are in this season, let's not struggle and whine but surrender to whatever His will may be for us. You may not leave a lineage to follow but be encouraged that like Daniel, childlessness does not mean uselessness in God's kingdom.

But men, even greater than Daniel, make *Jesus* the man you model your life after. He too walked this earth as a man, tempted in very way like us but without sin. He knew what it was like not to have a wife or children, and yet there is no way we can say he was foregoing any blessing in his life. Don't look to anyone or anything else to give you what only He can give you. Make him not just your example but your whole dependence and source of fulfilment.

CHAPTER 14

AN AWKWARD FIT

ONE AFTERNOON I BUMPED INTO a girlfriend from church at the supermarket checkout. We somehow got to chatting about church, and I asked her if she was planning to go the Bible study the next day.

"No, Jo, I went once but don't want to go back."

"Why?" I asked, a little disappointed. "It's been really good lately."

Her expression changed, revealing a hint of disapproval. "Well," she replied a little hesitantly, "the last time I just felt really awkward, like I just didn't quite fit. Most of the girls that go are all moms and well . . . well, I'm not, and if one more person asks me about kids . . ." Her answer trailed off. Normally such a gentle girl, it was unusual to see her even just a little annoyed.

Unfortunately, her sentiments are not so uncommon among young childless couples in general and women in particular within church. Repeatedly I hear the same concerns of these couples feeling they "just don't fit." Over and over again I hear the word "awkward" used when it comes to addressing the issues surrounding infertility within the church.

I do not recount this story to be critical of our churches but to highlight that such occurrences are often the normal experience of many couples within our congregations. I am the first to admit this is not an easy subject to broach without the risk of sounding condemning, which is definitely not my intention. My heart in writing this chapter is to help other members within a church body to better understand how those experiencing childlessness can feel and how we might work together to encourage and build one another up (Heb. 10:24–25). What I write here is not wholly our own personal experience but includes the opinions and experiences of different couples and individuals who are currently going through or who have been through this stage of infertility.

One of the main reasons so many childless couples feel like outsiders or like that square peg in a round hole is because being a parent seems woven into the identity of many of our friends in church. For them, much of their church life is dictated by the needs and requirements of their children. And that's okay. But we can't enter into that. While we can celebrate the kids and families that are there, we will never really understand how that works.

It is one thing to feel the pressure of being childless in our secular environment, but ironically this can feel even more intense within our church. Our Western church culture frequently elevates family life as the epitome of existence while simultaneously failing to recognize that for many, this is an impossible aspiration, leaving couples with a residual sense of being unfulfilled.

One can sit in the middle of a huge congregation and feel isolated. I am aware that for many struggling with infertility, church can become just one more struggle for a hurting couple to deal with. That place of closeness, understanding, and refuge has now become the very place that makes you feel your brokenness and loss just a little more keenly. Some of these most obvious difficult times include:

Mother's/Father's Day. These days can be difficult ones, I know. I question why we even celebrate them so publicly within church, often with a seeming lack of sensitivity. Mother's/Father's Day is a reminder to the infertile among us that they are unable to live out the reality of God's design for His people to bear children. Many times the presupposition is that even if they *aren't* parents themselves, they *have* parents to be thankful for and celebrate. This is also a painful day for many who are reminded that they do not have a loving, safe mother or father. Even within my own close circle of friends and family, I am all too aware of this. Not everyone, is, will be, or has a mommy or a daddy.

Children's Day or the Church Family BBQ. Um, you say *family* by which you mean kids, but I'm afraid I don't have one to bring. Or Christmas family celebrations. The constant references to children and family in the pastor's sermon illustrations.

Children/Baby Dedications. Perhaps one of the most difficult events for childless couples to witness. These can be painful. I shared my experience of how God transformed these moments for me in chapter 3, but I know for many others, these are dreaded mornings at church.

One of the reasons for all those in church—including the affected couples—may find it difficult to deal with these situations is because they are never exposed to the possibility of infertility before it happens. There may be no mention of childlessness in pre-marriage counseling classes and no obvious place or person within church to approach about these issues. During a chance meeting between my mom and a friend, the young woman began to tell her of the impact her infertility was having on her marriage, physical health, and emotional stability. After relating her story and choking back her tears, she ended by saying, "And you know what one of the worst things was? Not knowing who on earth we could talk to."

Her words filled my heart with sorrow. Other suffering couples had voiced similar feelings. This would be a good place for our churches to start helping these couples. Perhaps we need to begin to challenge the cultural norms in order to be more open and willing to break down these walls of silence.

THE SOUND OF SILENCE

Celebrity maternity guru, Rosie Pope, discussing her own struggle with infertility, said, "It's amazing to me that in Hollywood, it's okay to talk about drug addiction or divorce or cheating or whatever addiction you're going through, but it's not okay to talk about infertility."

Never mind Hollywood, her observation is exactly what most couples going through infertility experience; we just don't talk about it. Almost as if it's taboo, it seems everyone has real difficulty broaching this subject. People don't know what to say, whether that be the couple themselves or their friends and family or society at large. There is such a stigma associated with infertility that no matter the cohort we encounter, there seems to be that inevitable awkward silence.

This silence that exists in society in general permeates our church families too.

For many of us, our closest friends will be in church. Much of our social life and ministry or evangelistic work will include people from church. Most of our Bible study and gathered prayer and worship experiences will be as part of the church body. Indeed, church for many is a huge part of life.

At the same time, a couple's desperation for a baby will often be just as large a part of their lives, becoming, at times, all-consuming. A child of their own is all they want, and all they think about. Many of their days will be geared around planning how they can achieve this.

How strange it is then, that rarely do these two worlds meet. How is it possible that the two most important areas of our lives rarely seem to converge? We are involved in church and yet never utter a whisper about what is going on in our hearts. We don't grieve with others at the loss of an unborn child or the effect of the avalanche of hormones we just injected that very morning. We have to think of a new excuse each year for not attending the Mother's Day service or plan work for the day of the moms' Bible study. During this season, we are all too aware of the "sound of silence."

It's important that we don't place the entire fault for this lack of communication on one group or another. We acknowledge that, as struggling couples, we are as guilty of remaining quiet about our situation as our pastors, leaders, and church family.

Below are just some of the reasons that others have shared finding it difficult to openly discuss this subject, especially within a church environment. I have included a few reasons that a friend brought to my attention, some of which I hadn't considered. They are his observations as a church leader and so hopefully they will be helpful to other shepherds in understanding their congregations.

Sometimes, it's just too painful. We feel more protected if we just keep it to ourselves. One girl said that the first time they went through the IVF process, they let their family know and then very quickly wished they hadn't. Undertaking their second round of treatment, they decided to keep their decision to themselves. This was not because they did not have and appreciate their family's support but because they realized that the stresses of the treatment were too great to share. The lows were much lower than they had ever imagined and the hopes of their family much higher than they could deal with. Riding the roller coaster of emotions with their whole family was just too much. Can you imagine a larger church group knowing and the pressure that would add? In 1 Samuel 1, Hannah didn't want her family and friends to see the extent of her hurt, so she removed herself from the table after they had finished their meal and went to a place she felt safe enough to open her heart. Her husband's other wife was particularly cruel to Hannah, tormenting her about her infertility, and so it is perhaps not surprising that Hannah needed some space and privacy to confront these issues. Likewise, we too may need to find a "neutral" place and/or person to talk to and work through how these things are affecting our lives.

It's just difficult to trust your heart to someone and to believe that they'll "get it" and understand. Much of the time, we keep quiet because we are having enough bother just trying to understand and process our own feelings and circumstances; we just can't articulate them to anyone else.

The cause of our infertility, for whatever reason, is that our reproductive systems are not functioning as they should. I have covered this in detail in chapter 12, but what I often hear is that couples find it difficult to discuss their fertility issues in church because those not experiencing these problems find it awkward to talk about sex at a functional level. Whenever our bodies fail us in any other physical way that causes an illness or disability, there is often some form of support available because we realize that bodily abnormalities can affect the mental well-being of a person as well as the physical. I concede that for some this will just be too awkward a subject to discuss, but it's important to also be aware that this silence may leave a couple with no one to talk to about these things when much confusion exists.

Couples may fear that the personal becomes public, particularly within the life of a congregation where a general breakdown in trust has emerged that has made it very difficult to even take anyone into their confidence. These couples have difficult choices to make. They may feel their choice is either to suffer in silence or risk the embarrassment of public vulnerability or perceptions of disempowerment. For example, infertility can challenge that perception of being in control and self-determining, especially among those who live professional lives and are accustomed to controlling an environment in order to bring about change. In such cases, these individuals feel vulnerable about their inability to produce a child; and no matter how hard they try, they cannot produce a change in their circumstances. Their silence is in part due to their vulnerability, which is often perceived as weakness in a culture that promotes achievement. To regain power they will often consider any form of IVF treatment that will facilitate the production of a biological family. If they have evaded the ethical and indeed emotional implications of this, then they have likely resolved it is better to remain silent than to be challenged to reconsider.

I would also add to this point that for many professionally successful couples, there is often an element of shame felt when they have no other option than to undertake some form of ART. In a recent interview, supermodel Chrissy Teigen acknowledged that when she revealed she was attending a fertility clinic for help, she learned "that a lot of other people in your life are seeing these people and they have this shame about it." I would suggest this is also true for many within our affluent congregations.

Another reason that silence may persist is the notion that desires are in conflict with some biblical principles. For example, if the Scriptures encourage people to "seek first the kingdom of God and all these things will be added unto you," a number of responses may emerge. First, they may recognize that thoughts about childlessness are becoming ever more intrusive and as a result fear that such thoughts are eclipsing God as the object of their affections. In biblical terms, there's an intuitive sense that those longings contain an idolatrous element. This produces shame; the silence hides the shame and desire.

Sometimes there is no deep and meaningful reason why couples don't talk openly, and this can be attributed purely to personality. Stephan is one of the most open people I know. He wears his heart on his sleeve and will talk to anyone. I, on the other hand, am the complete opposite. Seems crazy to say this after writing this book, but I was one of the most private people you could ever meet, and with just about everything, not just our infertility. Not sharing our experiences with anyone in (or outside) church was just who I was. Some of us never feel a need to share our problems.

While I understand why *we* often remain silent, what confuses me more is why so little seems to be spoken about this subject by those in church leadership who are in the position of guarding, feeding, and caring for the flock.

JUST A LITTLE NOTE TO OUR SHEPHERDS

Pastor, if you are not already aware of the need for pastoral care concerning infertility within your church, then I would like to suggest you make a start. As the prevalence of infertility increases, so does the need for you to become familiar with the increasingly complex practical, scientific, and moral issues surrounding this area in order to guide and guard your flock wisely. Better that Christians come to you for advice than go looking for it in the world. Shepherds, these couples need you: they need to feel they can trust you to help with these concerns and that you have the confidence and knowledge to support them. This is not an easy task, I admit, but with infertility on the rise, this is a subject that you can no longer afford to ignore.

Upon asking a number of pastors in various countries why they felt infertility was addressed so little in our churches and why they found the subject difficult to tackle, I discovered that they all more or less came up with this same answers, some of which include the following:

"We just don't know what to say or how to broach the subject."

"I'm not even that sure what the Bible says about barrenness."

"We don't know what to say at all whether from the pulpit or personally."

"Not that many couples come to us in the first place with these issues so therefore we don't think they want us involved in the first place."

"How are we supposed to know if a couple is going through involuntary infertility or they are childless by choice? How are we supposed to ask?"

Without exception, all responded that much of the time they just found the whole topic plain awkward!

I do so sympathize somewhat with pastors in this. Oftentimes, it is very difficult to know whether a couple is struggling in this area and whether you should intervene. Even more difficult is determining whether there is secondary infertility or consented voluntary infertility. This may be even more difficult depending on the size of your church, but I would suggest there be some means available for couples to let their circumstances be known.

I also understand the feelings of inadequacy that many of you feel when trying to counsel people in this area. You may fear that a couple will automatically refuse your advice, especially if you have a family. You may assume they will think, "Who is he to give us advice? It's okay for him sitting there spouting when he has no idea really what we're going through." Few could blame you for feeling this way. It's true that at times you will not be able to answer their questions.

The truth is that I cannot answer them any better than you can. On many occasions, no one can give a hurting couple the answer they *want*, but you have the opportunity and the power to give them the answers they *need*. This is because the answers don't come from you or me but from Christ.

This can be a scary prospect. One pastor recently told me that when encountering people going through the pain of infertility, full of questions about why they couldn't get pregnant, he felt helpless. "How can I tell couples they need to work through the issue of idolatry in their lives when they so obviously want answers I can't give them? How can I be so insensitive to go there when they are obviously hurting deeply? What can I say when dealing with such emotions and longings in someone?"

Only a few weeks later, that same pastor spoke passionately about the power of speaking God's Word into someone's life. He reminded us that God's Word is more powerful and effective than anything we could ever say. His challenge to us was to endeavour to speak something of God's living words into someone's life that week. He truly believed that the power of the Scriptures was real and profound because of who wrote them and that those words were the means of transforming people's lives. I can only tell you the same thing. Go to God's Word for your answers and search the Scriptures to see what it has to say on this subject. When counseling these couples, you need to be both incredibly sensitive and bold at the same time!

Every encounter will most likely present different issues, and pastors/counselors will need to ask the Holy Spirit to guide them in how to respond to each individual couple. While everyone's experience is unique, let me alert you to a couple of areas of commonality that I have observed where you could help and support this young couple.

Depending on the stage of a couple's Christian walk and relationship with Jesus, these needs can vary.

It is highly likely that a couple wrestling with infertility will need support and prayer for their marriage. Also likely is that they will not ask for this help or share their intimate problems with you. Remember, chances are good they haven't been married for very long and may not feel comfortable sharing their concerns, especially if they don't know you very well. Again I think the example of Hannah (1 Sam 1) may be helpful here. Even though she never divulged the exact nature of her problem to Eli, she did allow him to see her heartbreak and following their brief encounter she "went her way and ate, and her face was no longer sad" (v18). Sometimes we don't need to share all the details of our struggles but to have a comforting, reassuring word can some days make all the difference to lift our spirits and dry our tears for that moment.

Therefore, no matter how awkward it feels, I would encourage you to get involved. The question of "should I intrude into someone's marriage or is this something that should be left private between a couple" is a difficult one to answer. But here's the thing: you can assume that, inevitably, infertility will have an impact on their marriage, albeit to a differing degree for each struggling couple. Often these couples are very young and find it very difficult to process what's going on inside their own heads, never mind trying to cope with their spouses.

During a panel discussion on the impact of infertility on a marriage, one common observation was that when many couples were going through treatment, it was almost as if they were in "survival mode" just to get through it. It wasn't until much later, after the treatment had ended and regardless of the outcome, that they started to realize the detrimental effect it had had on their marriage. Whether or not treatments resulted in a baby, in both scenarios the couples admitted they had to try and go back and fix their relationship.

Shepherds, knowing this information, wouldn't you agree that it's better to risk encountering a little awkwardness and perhaps confrontation in order to be a means of support for this couple, even if they don't realize they need it? Where you suspect infertility is an issue, wouldn't it be better to show them how to grow together through this experience than try to deal with the aftereffects? I have seen too many relationships in trouble. I believe one of the most powerful strategies our enemy uses is to break up Christian marriages and destroy our families, and if he can use infertility as a means of doing that, then he will!

Together, as a church family, we need to be vigilant about infertility. Shepherds, it's important to be aware that while infertility can be a means of drawing couples closer together, it can just as easily be a cruel crowbar to prise them apart. Even if the couple won't allow you in at this level, you'll know where your prayers for them need to be focused.

Another area that many couples struggle with is that of ART. While you perhaps may be inclined to approach the subject of infertility from any number of aspects, ART is nonetheless one of the most common topics of concern among Christian couples. Some couples have major concerns about these interventions, while others have no clue, and still others just need a little confirmation and reassurance. There is a plethora of "Christian" perspectives out there, and so I would encourage you to equip yourself with enough knowledge to teach and advise your congregation. There are moral questions that need to be considered as well as very practical ones. For example, some couples may encounter financial issues relating to their treatment, while others may receive it for free, depending on where they live. Some may have the opportunity to be treated in a Christian-based clinic, but others will receive advice from a secular facility. There may be polarizing theological and practical viewpoints within your congregation on these issues, so it is important you have some foundation for resolving these quandaries.

There is a strong need for support for those who have experienced the loss and grief of miscarriage. A far more open culture needs to be cultivated within church to allow these women and men to work through these experiences and be biblically guided and supported. During the course of a women's Bible study one evening, a random conversation arose about miscarriage. Within about 10 minutes, about every second or third woman had shared that they had suffered the loss of a baby and had struggled to deal with the aftereffects and grief. For most, it was the first time they had ever shared this part of their life with anyone, and all said they felt they would have benefited greatly by some form of support from within their church, even if that just meant they could be aware of and connect with others who had gone through the same turmoil. I know some couples who, having gone through miscarriages, are still struggling with bitterness toward their church years later because they felt the church ignored them, remaining silent in the face of their grief and acting as if nothing was wrong. They are still angry because they needed support that was never offered even though they were active members.

There seems to be a lack of understanding regarding the needs of such couples, though I suspect it's not due to a lack of love. Our fellow Christians just find the whole topic of infertility a bit awkward! It is important that the church be able to minister not only in love but also with a great deal of sensitivity.

INSENSITIVE LOVE

Our churches should be safe places for people to grow in trust with one another, a place where they can share their hearts without fear of being judged for speaking what may be shockingly honest. Sadly, this is often not what many experience. Sometimes there is a serious lack of sensitivity in the words spoken, even when well-intended. For example, after a prayer meeting one evening, a friend told me I was fortunate not to have any children. She further confided that she was praying for the Lord to close up her womb because she couldn't cope with more than the two kids she already had, and using contraception was such a hassle! Sounds crazy, right? But she was completely serious.

Later, another presumed-mature Christian woman shared that God kept giving her more and more kids so she could learn how to be a better mom.

Others I know have been deeply hurt by well meaning comments said to them when they miscarried, statements such as "oh, don't worry, you'll jump back in again in no time" or "well, at least you know you can get pregnant, so just keep trying till it happens again."

And then there's the favorite: "Well, have you prayed about it?" *What, are you kidding me?*

On the other hand, I completely understand that people search for something positive to say. They are scared of saying the wrong thing or being insensitive, and we childless couples need to give a lot of grace here too. We need to have a heart for forgiveness in this area because we know more than anyone that unless you experience infertility, you will have no concept of how it affects a person. A symbiotic relationship of grace and sensitivity between the two groups within the church is needed.

Pastors have an opportunity to teach their congregations how this should be and help everyone understand better how they can be sensitive and considerate to each other's needs and situations in life. I long to see a culture cultivated within our church families where the subject of infertility no longer remains taboo.

A FAMILY AFFAIR

For many Christians, the concept of being part of a church family remains precisely that: a concept. Often there is a disconnect between what we know about how a church should function in terms of being a family and the reality of that in our everyday lives. Do we really see each other as brothers and sisters in Christ? Do we, if we're really honest, live sacrificially for each other? Do we really live each day considering each other more significant than ourselves? (Phil 2:3-4) Do we as spiritual brothers and sisters have the same joy, same mind and same love as each other? (Phil 2:2) Are we really that close-knit of a family?

These questions are very convicting to my own heart because I believe our church lives would have a significant impact on those in need within our congregations if we had better understanding. Families are difficult, take a lot of work, and can be exhausting. They come in all sorts of messed up forms, but for the most part, because they are family, we are stuck with them and them with us. Is it any different when it comes to our church family? They too are often messed up. Yes, there's always the grumpy grandpa and the embarrassing uncle (or aunt in my case, as I'm so often told), the kind old granny, the irritable teenager, and the little cuties. But regardless, we have all been adopted into God's family. With Him as our Father and with His guidance, I think it is very possible that His kids might do things a little differently.

I believe it is possible to go from a place of feeling like an outsider to feeling completely included because the folks you worship with are indeed your brothers and sisters, your family. God has given us a natural desire to be part of a family and to love and raise children. Therefore, He may give us our church family and use us to serve the kids within our churches, to be a valuable part of their lives and influence for good.

However, it is also possible that He may have work that you wouldn't be able to do as a parent. Some time ago the Holy Spirit encouraged my heart when Stephan and I felt somewhat disconnected from our spiritual family and those we should have been close to. I did not lay the cause or blame for this perception at anyone's door, rightly or wrongly; it was just how we felt. The Holy Spirit reminded me of Daniel and how distinct he was not only from the Babylonians but also probably among his own kind. Not all the young men who had been taken into captivity refused to eat King Nebuchadnezzar's food. Only Daniel and his three friends abstained (Dan. 1). It was his uniqueness among his peers—the many taken into captivity with him

(1:6)—that prepared him for the work God had specifically for him to do. Daniel was still going to live and learn among his own countrymen from day to day, but within that community of people, God would give him a specific role. From the story of Daniel, we see that being slightly different isn't necessarily a disadvantage.

Sometimes, when we do not experience the typical paths in life, including having a family, that difference can leave us with a deep yearning for the "normal." Just to be the same as everyone else and experience the normal courses of natural life. However, it may just be that we have been given a different course for a specific reason because God has another purpose and strategy for our lives. Instead of being disheartened by the feeling of exclusion that infertility can bring, we can be encouraged by Daniel and know that while we may be different from those around us, God can use this for His glory. Even if Daniel was a bit weird, so what? God still had a place for him, and even if you feel different among your peers, He has a place for you too.

Whatever it is He had planned for us, God intends us to be a fully integrated part of His body, to love and serve those He has brought across our paths and into our lives.

Let Christ take you from that place of being an awkward fit to blending you into His family, where you will become connected with bonds formed and strengthened in Christ. Blood may be thicker than water but in our church families, can Spirit be thicker than blood?

CHAPTER 15

IT'S NEVER JUST "JUST . . ."

THERE ARE TWO EXTREMELY FRUSTRATING comments or questions that most couples struggling to conceive will hear at least once, if not many, many times.

The first is usually offered during the earlier stages of their journey: "*Just* relax, it'll happen when you least expect it. You need to stop stressing and *just* relax about it."

Ironically, when it becomes obvious that this isn't going to happen, the second response comes. "Why don't you *just* adopt?"

As an infertile couple, we know that for such decisions, there is no "just" about it! When it comes to the idea of adoption or fostering, a whole new set of questions and considerations comes into play. The conclusions are not and should not be arrived at with an attitude of it being "just."

Within each one of us, to a lesser or greater degree, is a God-given desire to nurture and mother a little one. Reinforced by our baby-bump society, the decision of whether to adopt can be very confusing and much more difficult for some than others.

Our desperation for a child may lead us to become foster or adoptive parents. This is a wonderful calling and one that delights the heart of God. You create a home for children who desperately need it, and you love and care for those young lives. It is a beautiful thing, displaying the gospel. It's an essential part of how our society operates. I love the fact that Jesus was an adopted kid, and the man accepting the role of his earthly father—Joseph—was, it would seem, just as honourable and obedient to God as Mary. You see, I don't think God makes mistakes about which family he places you in (Acts 17:26), whether that be natural or not. If you are a Christian couple considering fostering or adoption, it may be that God has those special children that are only supposed to be part of your family.

There are many means whereby a couple can become parents or be involved in raising children. As God brings these opportunities into your life, you will be enormously blessed. You will also experience some level of inevitable hardship along the way. But, it is no accident when children arrive in your life through this route. God doesn't "just" bring us together for no reason. No, He is the author of such things. Take confidence that while you may not have natural children, He may entrust other little ones to you. In many cases, these children do not have natural mothers and fathers and truly need you.

However, for many couples, this is not an option they want or have the ability to consider. I'm not convinced that anyone should judge a couple for choosing not to foster or adopt children, and no couple should feel guilty for not choosing to do so. There seems to be a perception right now within some Christian circles that every Christian family/couple should foster or adopt a child. The belief is that there are more Christian families than "homeless" children, and if we all did our part, this problem would be resolved.

I do not believe this to be the case and am more convinced that such lifestyles and life choices should be based on the fact that they are a *calling on your life* from God. Decisions of adoption, etc., shouldn't be made on a purely emotional response that can end up being as changeable as the wind.

Adoption doesn't always fulfil the desires of a couple's yearnings to produce their own natural children. I know couples that even after having adopted children are still working through and dealing with the effects of their infertility on their marriage, emotions, and physical health. It doesn't necessarily follow that the introduction of children leads to a cessation of issues surrounding a couple's infertility.

For some childless couples then, the option to undertake this role is rejected. They have no desire or conviction that they should be parents through such means. Friends, I wholeheartedly understand this perspective. As much as we wanted to be pregnant, neither Stephan nor I had a strong desire to foster or adopt children. Even when we realized it was highly unlikely we would ever have our own natural children, we did not feel a strong pull to adopt.

Straight off, many may think this a selfish attitude or that we don't really understand the importance or need to adopt. Ironically, I would suggest that we both have a vantage point in understanding how these things work.

Adopted as a newborn into a wonderful, young, Christian family, I grew up in a home that was always full of children. When I arrived, my parents already had two adopted sons who became my elder brothers. As a family we often discussed our adoptions. I was aware from a very young age that it was possible for a "mom and dad" to be unable to have their own biological children. Over the course of my young life, my folks were also foster parents to up to 60 kids, many of whom were pre-adoptive babies. Such experiences not only reinforced the reality of there being many childless couples in the world but I also became so accustomed to such things that I never regarded them as anything peculiar.

When I was around 11 years old, three new permanent additions were made to our family in the gift of adopted younger sisters. Like myself, they had all come from difficult circumstances. As our home came alive with the sound of crying babies and screaming toddlers, I started to question the fairness of who could or should have children against those who couldn't.

I was so very blessed with the family that God chose to place me in. For that, I will be forever thankful. He doesn't make mistakes. However, most adoptive kids ask many questions over their lifetime about their "natural roots." When we encounter one another, it's strange, but we tend to have a unique understanding and connection.

At university one evening, as Stephan and I sat in his dorm room looking through photos of his family, I asked him about his papa in one of the pictures.

"That's not my granddad," he replied. "That's my dad."

I was a little taken aback because the man in the photo looked really old, possibly even older than my own grandparents.

"Wow," I said, thinking I had stuck my foot in my mouth. "You definitely don't look like him. Your parents must have had you really late."

"Ummmm . . . actually, they did," he replied a little hesitantly. "My folks were married later in life, and the reason I don't look anything like either of them is because I'm adopted."

I started to laugh and thought how much of a coincidence this was. At first Stephan thought I was laughing because I found the situation awkward—until I told him I was adopted too. We laughed together then and in that moment I believe we formed another bond that would affect, in part, how we would live our lives in the following years. Both of us knew first-hand what it meant to not only be adopted kids but also what we meant to our adoptive parents.

So why, when we both understand the need for adoption and have been so blessed through it, didn't we believe God called us to the same purpose?

I am not sure I can answer that. These are difficult topics. Some of the most Christ-like couples I know include childless ones who chose not to adopt or foster children. We cannot judge any couple's decision, but if their desire for a family could be solved by a "just," then you can be sure it would.

Sometimes, God had His own way of bringing children into one's life to love and care for when least expected. That is exactly what happened to us. Within a very short span of time, our two little nephews came to live with us. Our lives changed overnight, and the "shock to the system" was no little one. We went from working crazy busy jobs to wondering what the heck to put in a packed lunch box! The little convertible sports car had to be replaced by a "clunky" family car with car seats! Saturday mornings were now spent standing frozen at the edge of the rugby field and afternoons sitting at some fishing spot. I had to begin learning how to cook (I use that term loosely) and blew up more eggs and burnt more dishes than were edible. I even tried boiling potatoes without water and wondered why it wasn't working. I kid you not, our heads were fried!

From then on, our house became a place where kids congregated. On the majority of our weekends, our home was full of kids that we got to love on and share a little joy with. Some of these children had no daddy, so we held many of their birthday parties, took them with us on summer trips, helped them with their education, and gave them cuddles when they were needed.

This was definitely not the life I had envisioned for myself, but what an honour and privilege it has been to be involved in the lives of so many kids and teenagers! However, though we are Aunty and Uncle to "our" boys and have witnessed first-hand the need for couples to step into children's lives, we still do not feel a calling on us to extend our family.

Whatever it is that God has called you to in life, whether or not that includes parenting, make seeking after Jesus your first priority. I know this can sound like a pat, biblical answer, but it is nonetheless true. When you endeavour to walk close to Jesus, listen for His voice, and ask Him to give you an obedient spirit and heart to serve, then many of these difficult decisions will start to make sense. His word and the counsel of spirit-filled men and women will guide you as you traverse this season of your life. I know only too well that God can change your plans right under your nose. *Just* ask Him to prepare you for whatever and whomever He decides to entrust to your care.

CHAPTER 16

WHEN THE TIDE GOES OUT

IT WOULD BE EASY TO assume that women who have passed the age of being physically able to conceive no longer struggle with the emotional aspects associated with barrenness. However, from my observations, this is an untrue correlation. Indeed, a whole new spectrum of emotions may come into play. Evidence of lingering heartache is reflected in a few of the responses I have heard from women who have reached that stage in their lives when their physical childbearing years have passed, including these:

> One of the greatest regrets of my life was never having children.

> The most difficult time of my whole experience of infertility was when I realized my body was no longer biologically able to have children.

> Going through menopause was the hardest time for me. The reality hit me that I would never give birth. This is still the worst period of my life of barrenness because now there is no going back, and any hope I might have had is gone.

I admit this is a difficult chapter to write because I'm personally not there yet and therefore cannot fully relate to the thoughts and feelings of these women. However, it is among those I have felt most compelled to write and consider one of the most important. My heart aches when I read these sentiments and hear the pain in the voices of those who are not grieving the loss of something they had and then lost but of what they never possessed in the first place and now never will. A deep sense of finality is felt. For many, menopause not only spells the cessation of their physical reason for "being" as a woman but also represents the end of their lifelong hopes and dreams. What a terrible place to be, to encounter a finality to your perceived physical and emotional purpose combined with a dashed hope in the latter stages of your life. This is especially sad and troubling to me because I do not believe it is God's desire that anyone should live in that state of emotional turmoil of regret and dissatisfaction. To remain there would surely be a nightmare and I suspect is borne out of a lifetime of experiencing continual disappointment, building up resentment, and harbouring the possession of a misplaced hope.

While we considered this issue of misplaced hope in a previous chapter, it may perhaps be important to take a fresh look at it again for this particular season of your life. If your hope was placed in there being a "maybe baby," then where is your hope now, if you still have any? Has it failed you along with your aging biological body?

Ladies, with the deepest of respect to the generations above me, I want to encourage you that if you are one of these grieving women, there is still time to find a new source of joy and fulfilment in your life that's even better than anything you dreamed of before. As a woman in my thirties, I cannot write this chapter as one sharing in your experience, and so I want to write to you from a younger woman's perspective and share with you what God has laid on my heart for your generation now.

First, I have too often noticed a common misperception among many older people in church that they feel they do not have much to offer or anything of great import or value to impart to the generations coming up after them. How often I hear remarks like "It's all about the young ones; after all, they are the future of the church," or "What do we know? The younger generation has its own way of doing things now. It's not our time anymore."

I couldn't disagree more.

I am telling you, couples of my generation and even younger realize as we get older that not only do we need you, we are crying out for your help. We desperately need you to come alongside us, hold our hands to teach us and guide us through these difficult times in our lives. All of you who have been walking in the faith far longer than any of us have so much wisdom and life experience that we value and crave. While I don't believe we need to go through the same struggles to be able to help one another, for those of you who find yourselves in the category of being an older childless couple in the church, oh my, what a distinct treasure you are to us! What a God-given opportunity you may have to touch lives and to tend to the wounds of members of your church family in ways no one else can. The cry of my heart is that you do not let these opportunities pass because you feel embarrassed or ill-equipped. We need you! We need your biblical wisdom, knowledge, and understanding. We need people we can look up to who have a deep strength and quiet grace that makes us think you are held together with invisible rods of spiritual steel. Your insight has come from years of friendship with Christ that we admire and are inspired by. When we look at you, we see the grace of God shining out of your life. Seeing God's hand at work in your life strengthens our faith in believing He is working in us too.

I truly believe this kind of mentoring can happen between us today because I see its power in the lives of a special little group of very ordinary yet extraordinary individuals in the Bible. I was so struck by how the influence of an older woman had a profound effect on one much younger. Just take a few moments now and read the whole of Luke chapter 1 and delight your heart anew with the happenings and characters within the narrative.

The relationship between Elizabeth and Mary in this story is especially beautiful. These are two women who find themselves in the same position while being poles apart in their season of life. Elizabeth is old, having gone through menopause many years before. Mary is not yet married and still a virgin. Neither of these women had any thought of becoming pregnant at that time of their lives, one because her time had passed, and the other because her time had not yet come. However, now they are both expecting children that were conceived by the power of the Holy Spirit, going against everything that nature would dictate is possible.

Often when we read or hear this passage taught, we focus on Mary's experiences and assume that her responses, especially in her conversation with Gabriel, are borne out of her exclusive relationship with and understanding of God. That in part is true, but I suspect that the presence of Elizabeth in Mary's life holds far more import and influence than we might first perceive.

When considering Mary's words and actions, sometimes we skip straight to when she says to the angel, "Behold, I am the servant of the Lord; let it be to me according to your word" (v38). But this is not her initial response to his declaration. We need to step back and look more closely at her insecurities.

Understandably, Mary's first reaction was to ask Gabriel, "How can this be?" She was fully aware of the biological functioning of her body. She cannot fathom how she could be pregnant, and I think it is very telling how Gabriel addresses the question of her heart and lips. He begins by explaining how this whole pregnancy was going to occur— "the Holy Spirit will come upon you, and the power of the Most High will overshadow you; therefore the child to be born will be called holy – the Son of God" (v35).

I don't know about you, but if that had been me, I don't think I would have understood the explanation. Mary's mind must have been reeling at the knowledge that she was talking to an angel, especially with the heavy stuff Gabriel was laying on her. I know I'd have asked him to repeat himself at least a few more times before I even got the gist of his message. But it was the second part of his answer that I think could have elicited Mary's submissive response. She could relate to and connect with that part of his answer because it was about a woman she knew and understood. "And behold your relative Elizabeth in her old age has also conceived a son, and this is the sixth month with her who was called barren. For nothing will be impossible with God" (v36-37).

I'm inclined to think that it was only after the angel told her about Elizabeth that Mary had the confidence and trust to declare her own servanthood toward God. Is it possible that her awareness of God's supernatural hand in Elizabeth's life made it easier to accept that the same God who could circumvent the biological impossibilities in Elizabeth could do the same in her body? I could be persuaded to believe this was so. Mary had probably known Elizabeth for the duration of her young life. Recognizing her as a woman who walked with God, Mary took confidence in following Elizabeth's example by submitting herself to God's will.

In contrast to Mary's youthful questioning, Elizabeth's response is one of quiet confidence and acceptance that came from a lifetime of walking in friendship and dependence on God. "Thus the Lord has done for me in the days when He looked on me, to take away my reproach among people" (v25). I suspect this was an aspect of her character that Mary had witnessed before and was one reason why she was now drawn to Elizabeth and wanted to be near her to share what God was doing in her life. So in the days following her encounter with Gabriel, Mary packed a bag and went to visit Elizabeth and Zechariah.

Mary didn't choose to be with this older woman because she thought Elizabeth would have the best pregnancy or parenting tips out there. No, these women now had not only a natural connection but a deep, spiritual one. As much as their years separated them, they were bonded by their servant's hearts and love toward God. They were both living through the process of God working a miracle in their lives, day after day for nine months. Every other woman they knew had experienced the natural process of pregnancy, but for these two, their pregnancies were supernatural. I imagine their time together was spent in conversation about and worship of their God, being full of wonder of who He was and what He was bringing about in their lives.

In their connection together, we can see how important this older woman Elizabeth is and how she is just as much part of this story as the younger Mary. Isn't it remarkable that not only was this godly woman chosen to be the mother of John the Baptist, but that God waited until she was old before it happened? Could it have been that the purpose for Elizabeth's barrenness all these years was so that now she was best placed to be able to help Mary when Christ was due to be born?

God knew what Mary would experience in the coming months and the pressure she would face from those around her, and He chose this mature woman of incredible spiritual character to be the mother of Christ's forerunner as well as the friend and guide to the mother of His Son. Elizabeth was there to strengthen and support Mary right from the time when Mary heard from Gabriel. Who better could Mary have had to encourage her? God's timing and the methods He uses to bring key people into our lives is perfect.

As you think on this story, I want to ask those of you who may have remained childless or have struggled throughout your life with infertility to consider rethinking God's purpose for this season of your life. Could it be that you have been placed in your town or church for the specific reason of encouraging, comforting, and building up younger women in their faith and worship of God?

Elizabeth's story was a huge source of encouragement to Mary. It appears that after having spent time in the company of Elizabeth, Mary went from a place of questions and confusion to one of praise and worship to God her Saviour. This is demonstrated in one of the most famous passages in the Bible, known as "Mary's Song," where Mary so beautifully expresses her heart of worship toward God. Her words though, only come subsequent to the words of encouragement, praise, and worship spoken by Elizabeth. It's not a stretch to believe the time Mary spent time in the company and presence of Elizabeth had a huge impact on her and the words that she would utter. Is it possible that we have "Mary's Song" not solely because of her personal relationship with God but also in part because of her connection with Elizabeth? I believe there are young women all over the world who are crying out for relationships like that in our church families. Please, older women, do not underestimate your strength, wisdom, and influence for good on younger women. You can help answer their questions, stem their confusion, and lead them to a place of worship and praise to the same "God, *our* Saviour."

Perhaps you feel this is too high a calling, that you aren't worthy or can't see yourself as an Elizabeth. I want to humbly challenge you that you may indeed be just the exact person to fulfil this task.

Zechariah, Elizabeth's husband, was also present in the house and witness to all the goings on. Surely he, being a priest and having greater biblical knowledge and learning, would be the best person to try to make sense of God's hand in all these happenings and be the respected person to counsel and advise Mary. But he was unable to speak for the entire period of Elizabeth's pregnancy and doesn't appear to have had a role in Mary's story at all. Instead, it was Elizabeth who spoke into Mary's life and had the effect that she did.

Sometimes, we make the same assumptions and think these conversations are best left to professional counselors or pastors. After all, they are the guys we look up to for spiritual instruction and direction for applying the Scriptures to our lives. Don't even begin to think like this! I prefer the wisdom of an Elizabeth, an older woman full of the Holy Spirit, a woman who reveals evidence of God working in her life. I don't want counsel borne out of what someone in a pastoral role thinks should be said. Rather, we need people to speak a living word from the Lord into our lives. We need those who will walk through this season of life with us, pray with us, and be instrumental in turning our hearts toward Christ so that together, like Mary and Elizabeth, our hearts and voices are knit in wonder and worship for Christ.

My heart is thrilled even as I write these words and imagine these sorts of connections and relationships being made within the family of God. I know they sound almost too idealistic to be a reality within every Christian community, but I believe they are possible. Most of us are ordinary women living ordinary lives within ordinary towns and cities. Yet we have opportunities to establish God-appointed relationships with each other. That has the potential to change our lives, our churches, and our wider communities. Do you not see the explosive potential you as older women have to create and be a part of a spiritual legacy that transcends any natural one we could ever hope to establish?

Therein lies one of the most fundamental questions of our Christian journey: what legacy do I want to leave? Whose name is it that I want to be associated with or be remembered for? Is it my own earthly family name or is there another name above that, one that is more important to be held up and honoured? Most definitely there is! "Therefore God has highly exalted him and bestowed on him the name that is above every name, so that at the name of Jesus every knee should bow" (Phil. 2:9-10a). What a privilege and joy to be associated with the name of Jesus and represent Him first.

This inspirational attitude of heart can be clearly seen in the story of Elizabeth and Zechariah. In their culture, names carried huge significance and would often describe and indicate the desire of the parents for their children. Therefore, Elizabeth and Zechariah's friends and family expected they would, and should, name their new baby "Zak junior" after his daddy, for the precise purpose of carrying on the family name. Instead, this couple called him *John* just as God had requested, because their son's purpose in life was not to exalt his earthly father's name but the Son of his Heavenly Father. His legacy was to lift up the name of Jesus!

By naming their son *John*, they acknowledged that there was something more important than carrying on their own name. I wonder if these godly parents knew that their own natural line would die with John. John's life was not to include a wife and family of his own. He had another calling and purpose: he was going to draw people to Jesus. He was to establish a completely different kind of legacy and my, what a legacy he left behind. Indeed, Jesus was later to say of him, "among those born of women none is greater than John" (Luke 7:28a).

Imagine Christ speaking words with even just a hint of such sentiments about you or me. Does that not thrill your heart like nothing else? Maybe, like John, you have no human lineage to leave behind, but what a spiritual legacy you could leave. You could be involved in the lives of God's people and unbelievers in ways that would turn your and their worlds upside down because you have chosen to lift *His* Son up to the world and not your own.

I am convinced that you who are both mature in the faith and in life have a work and a ministry that cannot be carried out by another group of people. Please don't ever think you are past it or have little or nothing to offer. It may seem to you at times that the younger generations have all the energy, drive, and vision. You may even wonder if God could really speak to you now or give you a fresh insight and work to do.

The story of Elizabeth and Zechariah dispels any doubt that this could happen in your life. At the beginning of the story, we read that Elizabeth is filled with the Holy Spirit. The presence of the Holy Spirit in those moments gave her the words to speak to the mother of Jesus that not only demonstrated her own humility and love for God but also had a profound effect on the heart of Mary and most likely contributed to the production of one of the most beautiful songs of worship in the Scriptures.

A little later in the story, after John was born, it was Zechariah's turn to be filled with the Holy Spirit (v67). Under the influence of the Spirit of God, he spoke great words of vision and prophesy about how his son would lift up the name of the Saviour. In both instances when this couple were filled with the Holy Spirit, their hearts were taken up with Christ and the legacy and work that He was to fulfil. Never did they indicate a desire for their own name to be carried on. In verses 67–79, Zechariah seemed amazed that his son John was going to have the privilege of being a part of creating the legacy the Messiah would establish.

This is a couple, full of the Holy Spirit, who are both OLD. The power of the Holy Spirit is not just for the young and dynamic. It is available to all ages, to give us a vision and equip us to perform a work that only we can do.

Go after it, no matter your age or stage in life, and I guarantee you will see fruit for your labour. I cannot begin to tell you the effect it will have on me and many others if our lives are touched by an Elizabeth or Zechariah. We want to be part of your legacy, that one day we will be able to share and celebrate together in heaven.

The righteous flourish like the palm tree . . .

They still bear fruit in old age;

They are ever full of sap and green,

To declare that the Lord is upright.

~Psalm 92:12–15

For more information about
Joanna Graham
&
The Inconceivable Truth
please visit:

www.theinconceivabletruth.com

For more information about
AMBASSADOR INTERNATIONAL
please visit:

www.ambassador-international.com
@AmbassadorIntl
www.facebook.com/AmbassadorIntl

www.ingramcontent.com/pod-product-compliance
Lightning Source LLC
Chambersburg PA
CBHW071022280326
41935CB00011B/1458